THE STORY THAT MADE US STRONGER

IRIS MARCH

This book has always been dedicated to the real Katie: my brave, fierce sister Meg.
Katie's story mimics much of what Meg went through in her battle against Hodgkin's lymphoma and the early life of my sweet nieces.
I'm proud to be your sister, Meg. You still amaze me. With all my love.

Katherine is Meg's middle name and so was an easy choice for her character. Meg's niece was also named Katie, her husband's brother's daughter. Little Katie passed away as an infant and is sorely missed and deeply loved. This story also honors her memory.

THE RUNNER

Connor Jackson

I'd run past it probably a thousand times.

An especially windy thunderstorm had covered my regular paved running trail with slippery leaves, twigs, and a few larger limbs on a late August afternoon. As I was running the trail, avoiding the more slippery sections, a door that I'd never noticed before was ever-so-slightly crooked, leaving it ajar. Mind you, I was running when I caught this dark shadow next to the door in the corner of my eye, and I almost tripped. Instead of hitting the ground, I sidestepped and took that moment to stop, pretend to tie my shoe and adjust my socks, and push my sweaty brown hair out of my eyes. I refused to be one of those guys with a man bun, but maybe I just needed to get a new haircut.

As I was messing with my shoes, I looked up at the building. It was small, probably only ten feet long by ten feet wide, a red-brick structure with a huge pole an inch away from it that was taller and thicker than any nearby telephone poles. At the tip of the pole was a piece of metal, strapped on and reaching even farther into the sky. There was a rusted chain-link fence around the building, with a few small trees and weeds within it. You could tell at one point that green plastic had been wrapped around the links, but it was long gone. The building was about fifty feet away from the trail, with plenty of trees between it and me, including a huge tulip poplar that I often noticed while running, and a bunch of maples. Breaking up the brick on the west side of the building, facing up the trail, was a wooden door with no window, adorned only by a worn doorknob. And now the hinges seemed to have broken a bit, the wood warped and pulling away from the frame about half an inch.

I was kneeling and staring for too long. A woman wearing blue sunglasses and walking a dog that looked like Lassie gave me a bit of a sideways look. I adjusted my shorts and stood up to continue running, with a lot more on my mind.

———

AFTER I GOT HOME from my three-miler, I plopped down on my couch with some water. My feline room-mate, Pumpkin Muffin, plopped down next to me. We're definitely both ploppers. He's a fat orange tabby who doesn't like to sit on laps. My niece named him during a stint when she ate pumpkin muffins for breakfast every day. I couldn't argue: he's totally pumpkin color. We lived in a condo with a walking path right from my patio to the

Park District trail I was just running on. The two-bedroom condos in the same development were cheaper, but this was the only one for sale with the path, so I went for the three bedroom. I guess I was also optimistic five years ago that my relationship status would change more rapidly. It's only ever been Pumpkin and me living here, other than a few houseguests and sleepovers with my nieces.

"Pumpkin, I can't stop thinking about this building." He looked at me, asking with his eyes for me to continue. He was massaging both the afghan my cousin Stephanie had knitted for me and the blue microfiber of my couch with his front paws. Pumpkin was still fixing me with his kitty stare, and I knew not to pet him while he was doing his massaging thing.

"I mean, I go past it every time I run the trail, but this time the door was open," I told him. He looked interested, which made me want to blurt out everything. "It's an old, abandoned building that has always been really run-down. And now even more. I have no idea what it was or why it's still standing." By this time, Pumpkin had found a new spot on the couch and was curling up, ready for a nap, his attention no longer on my story.

"I really want to know what's inside," I said. "I don't know that I'm the breaking-and-entering kind of guy, though." I ran my hand down his back and tail and stood up. I poured the rest of my water into my wilting snake plant in the hallway as I made my way into the bathroom to take a shower. "Not that kind of guy," I repeated to myself.

THE STEM CELL REPLACEMENT WARD

Connor Jackson

The next morning, at the start of my shift on the stem cell replacement ward, I was daydreaming about what might be inside the building. Why was it so small? What was the huge pole for? Did it connect to something inside the tiny room? Was there a dirt floor? Had animals invaded, and were they living in there now? Was there a basement?

After saying hello to coworkers, I looked over the patient charts. Then I set off to check in on my first patient of the day, Katie.

"Good morning, Katie." I said as I entered her room, knocked on her door, announced my arrival and entered. This was her third day on the floor, and she was still feeling about as healthy as she had when she arrived. We jumped right into her daily weigh in.

"How was your night, Connor, my man?" Katie asked as I made notes on my laptop. Katie had shoulder-length, curly blonde hair and the most decked-out room I've ever seen in my six years working on this ward. The rooms are large, as comfortable as they can be for a hospital. She had brought her own bright-pink quilt and pillows, had strings of lights up and pictures plastered everywhere. One entire wall was covered with photos of amazingly cute kids. Katie and her husband, Travis, had a boy who would be three in a few months and twin girls who were just born five months ago, when Katie had full-on Hodgkin's lymphoma. This lady had a lot to live and fight for. She was there to get a stem cell transplant to make sure she never had lymphoma again. It would take three weeks, and her health would really fade in the next few days as we killed all her white blood cells.

"I went on a run and played some video games. I was in the mood for Indian. Well, I'm always in the mood for Indian, so I made some aloo gobi," I said. "Kind of boring." I took her temporal temperature and made another note.

"Not as boring as my night. I'm already totally done with watching TV and movies." She was twirling her hair. "I miss my little people so much."

Katie's procedure is called "stem cell replacement," but some use the term "bone marrow transplant." A week before she was admitted, we harvested a lot of Katie's blood to use later. (And when I say "we," I mean another department in the hospital.) The lab spun down the blood to harvest her stem cells. While she was staying on my ward, we were giving her longer, higher doses of chemo to kill all her white blood cells and lower her absolute neutrophil count (ANC). Neutrophils are the white-blood-cell infection fighters that we pay the most attention to. We were killing her immune system in order to build it back up later. Lymphoma patients often develop leukemia later in life, and these treatments would ensure that she would not. After her numbers were at zero, we'd transfuse her stem cells back into her body, and it would recover fairly quickly. Katie was a fighter, and we were expecting better-than-normal results. Most patients with Hodgkin's lymphoma go on to live healthier lives than before having cancer, even getting fewer colds. Not to say that the next six months would be a walk in the park. Katie's immune system would still be compromised, and everyone around her would need to treat her system like that of a newborn. She'd get the same vaccines that infants get again. But a year from now, Katie would be a new woman, a super-healthy mama to her miracle-baby twins and little man.

Katie had been the main caregiver for her kids before she was diagnosed with cancer. It's hard to pull a mom away from her kids, I know. Her husband would take a month off work after she returned home to care for her and those kids full time. Right now he wasn't able to visit as often as the rest of her family. There are only two hospitals in the state that provide this treatment, and he and Katie lived more than an hour away so Travis wasn't able to visit as often as he would have liked while working full time.

"You're video-chatting with the fam every night, right?" I asked. "After Travis gets home from work, aren't you on the TV the entire night until the kids' bedtime?" I was thinking of telling her about the building because I couldn't get it out of my mind. Katie knew the drill of the vitals I needed to take. She adjusted her shirt sleeve without me asking so I could take her blood pressure. Katie didn't wear our hospital gowns, opting for comfortable clothes instead. I don't know why no one else on our ward had thought of that. She said that it made her feel more at home at the hospital.

"Yeah, but PJ isn't so into talking to me over the TV. He doesn't really get it," she sighed, and changed the subject. "I can't wait to go on a run again. I used to run 5Ks and some triathlons, you know. I ran a marathon relay once. Your half-marathon is going to be great. I'm proud of you for training so hard."

"I hope you're right." Sometimes it's weird to get encouragement from a person so sick, someone you should be encouraging instead. "My half is only four weeks away. I'm feeling good about it so far." I did the blood draw, and Katie waited for me to finish. It's hard to continue a conversation while drawing someone's blood.

"What's your long run going to be this week, then? Where are you running?" she asked, as if the conversation had never paused.

"Eleven miles this Sunday. I go on the Park District trail near my house." I took a deep breath. "And there's an abandoned building on the trail I was on last night that I can't get out of my head."

"Oh, yeah? 'Abandoned building' sounds exciting!" I was cleaning up all my supplies by this time, and I could tell that Katie, like Pumpkin, was interested in the building, too.

"It's a tiny brick building, and now the door is kind of

falling off its hinges," I told Katie. Her eyes widened as I described building, fence, and pole. I was glad her attention span was longer than a cat's.

"Well, can you get into it? What's in there?"

"I keep thinking that I want to pry the door open, but there are always people on the trail. It's a busy place," I said, typing everything into my computer.

"You have to try! Where is it?" Katie got out her phone and was looking at her maps app. I found my little town of Hawthorn Heights in northeastern Ohio and the trail, but the building wasn't on the map, so I couldn't point to it directly.

"Well, I want to know what's in it," Katie said in a determined voice. "Because we all want to find something amazing, some treasure in old, abandoned places. That's what we expect."

The attending doctor came in to talk to Katie about the chemotherapy treatment she was getting that day. I slipped away with my computer and blood vial, thinking of treasure and amazing finds.

Later that day, I stopped in for yet another vitals check and to change Katie's chemo bag. We inject chemo meds via syringe into the IV port Katie had on her right shoulder. She was about to get her third chemo bag of the day.

"Hey, Connor," Katie said, gesturing at the older couple standing near her bed, "my mom and dad are here. Phil and Lydia."

"Nice to meet you," I said. "I'm Connor, Katie's normal daytime nurse during her stay here. I just need to take some more vitals. Every two hours, you know!"

Her mom, who also had curly hair, was adding to the messages of encouragement on Katie's windows with a dry-erase marker.

"Her numbers are where you want them to be?" Phil asked me, rubbing his fingers over his silver mustache.

"We want those white blood cells at zero by Sunday. The ANC should be near the bottom, too. Your daughter is strong, though. Her blood is putting up a fight," I said with a smile, and turned to Katie.

"So, how are you feeling? Itchy? Any swelling or burning? Do you feel hot anywhere? What about a headache or upset stomach?" Katie shook her head at each question. She had a history of allergic reactions to some meds, and we were keeping a close watch on her, asking extra questions. We kept a crash cart down the hall to make sure we had supplies on hand in case of any negative reactions. Her parents watched our back-and-forth closely. I took notes on my computer cart.

"Well, we were just leaving," Phil announced after watching me for a minute, and Lydia finished her message. They exchanged goodbyes with their daughter before I got my needle ready.

Phil clapped me on the shoulder and said, "Take care of her." I assured them both that I would. Adult or not, having your child in the hospital for any length of time is hard. I knew how much his family has been through this year with Katie's pregnancy and her cancer diagnosis.

"I'm so excited about this abandoned building! It's like we're solving a mystery!" Katie whispered to me after they left.

"I'm excited, too! It's cool to have someone to be excited with!" I whispered back.

Katie and I saw each other every few hours during that shift but didn't talk about the building again because she always had visitors or another medical professional attending to her treatments.

3

THE GOLF COURSE MANAGER

Katie Brandt

After Connor left for the day, I was amped up as I always was after chemo. My body was worn out and aching, but my mind wouldn't stop. I tried to take a nap but couldn't find sleep, even with the blinds closed and all the lights off. I just kept thinking about my kids, having conversations with them in my head about why I was away from them. I was doing this stem cell replacement ordeal for them: so that their mommy wouldn't get leukemia later in their lives. I'd promised that I'd never leave them.

No matter the time of day, I usually had a hard time getting to sleep in this bed, in this hospital room. I dragged myself across the room and found my computer. After I settled back into bed, I searched Google Maps and found the area that Connor had pointed out before. His excitement was contagious, and now I wanted to know more about that building too. I saw the golf course and some of the trail through the trees on the satellite images. Once I clicked on the road view, I could see the building itself that Connor was talking about. It really looked old despite the grainy picture, yet somehow familiar. I wondered if I had driven past it before. I looked up the golf course and poked around their website and then the Park District's website.

"Someone has to know something!" I said to myself. There was a list of historical buildings that the Park District managed, but nothing about one being on or near that golf course. After twenty minutes of not finding anything to give me a single answer, I decided to just call the Park District itself. Why not? It was still only 3:45; they'd be open. I dialed the Administration Office down-town first.

"Hello, Park District Administration Office. This is Tammy. How can I help you?" Her spiel sounded very rehearsed and overly chipper.

"Hi, Tammy. My name is Katie. I'm a resident of Hawthorn Heights and was wondering if you guys can tell me more about an interesting building that sits along a trail I frequent. I have a bet with my friend about who can find out info about it fastest." I could really turn on the charm when I needed to, even when I didn't feel well. Call it a gift. When you used a person's name and told them they were doing you a favor, they wanted to help most of the time. I was also good at seeing everyone as a person, not just someone in my way. I knew everyone had their own thing going on and tried to respect that.

"What an interesting request, Katie!" Tammy exclaimed. She was really excited about this, too, and we were both name users. I hoped she didn't see through my charm. "Let me see if I can find it on our maps."

I told her where the building was located.

"Yes, I see it here, Katie."

"Great!" I said, excited that it was so easy to find out more about it. I'd always believed in the power of a phone call and some kindness.

"I'm sorry, Katie. There's no further information that I see beyond that it is on our map." Tammy might have been going overboard on the name using, but at least she was feigning disappointment. "I can transfer you to our Architectural Office. They know the most about our built environment, after all."

"I'd appreciate that. Thank you so much," I said. After she politely gave me the phone number she was transferring me to, I got on the phone with another gate-keeper, this time, Calvin.

He actually said the exact thing Tammy did: "What an interesting request, Katie!" I almost laughed. He continued, "Let me see what I can find. I'm going to put you on hold for just a moment while I ask a few people." Hold music came on, and I waited. Calvin returned after three minutes and said he was sorry it was taking so long and could he take down my number or leave me on hold longer. I told him I'd wait, but after another four minutes, I hung up with a new plan. I felt bad leaving Calvin hanging, but he was leaving me hanging, too, after all.

I called the Peregrine Falcon Golf Course directly next. This time, a young man named Victor answered the phone in a rather bored voice.

"Victor! Just the man I was hoping to talk to. This is

Katie. I live near your golf course and am interested in a small building near the adjoining trail. I bet you know all about it. What can you tell me, Vic?" I realized I was totally pretending to live in the same house as Connor. It was kind of weird, but a citizen gets more traction than someone who is out of town.

I had obviously taken Victor by surprise. "Me? You were looking for me? What's your last name? How do you know people call me Vic?" Maybe I had been a bit too forward with this guy. Someone must have drilled him too hard about stranger danger as a child.

"I'm sorry, Victor. It was just a hunch. I had an Uncle Vic who was really great." I wished I could pat him on the shoulder or something.

"Well, most people call me Vic . . ." he said hesitantly.

"I was just calling to learn more about that little building near the trail. I figured a young, enthusiastic guy like you would know about it," I said. Here's another secret about people: you can talk characteristics into them. Calling Victor enthusiastic was not something I was doing because I thought he was enthusiastic. It was because I wanted him to be.

"Oh. I know the building you're thinking of. It's kind of falling apart, right?"

"It really is," I agreed. "And if I were in high school, I'd really want to get into it."

He laughed, loosening up. "It's, like, super old. But it's locked up tight."

"It is?" I asked quickly, trying to show my own enthusiasm as much as possible, but letting him lead the conversation.

"Yeah, I tried to get in last year with Chuck, but together we couldn't bust it. I guess you know high schoolers. We've been thinking about getting in there for years," Victor told me, sounding impressed with himself.

"Man, Victor! You couldn't get in? But do you know what it was for originally? Or how the Park District uses it?" I asked, hoping he'd know something more.

"I really don't think we use it at all. Our manager, Leah, would know more, though. I don't think she's in a meeting or giving a lesson or anything. Let me see if she's in her office. Just a minute." More hold music. It didn't dissuade me, though. I had cracked this gatekeeper, and he was a good guy. I really do think that all people really are good deep down.

The hold music cut off, and a sweet voice said, "This is Leah Alger." With charm in full swing, I told her my tale.

"It's a really unusual little building. I've been trying to find out more about it myself," Leah said.

"You have?" I asked, almost dumbfounded.

"It's been there forever, but it's not well documented," she told me. "I tried to ask our architectural group. They knew about it but weren't interested in it at all. It did not surprise them that there weren't digital files on it. I had to dig around at our Park District map room to find any information. I keep wondering if some old-timers in town would know more about it." What a good idea. I wondered if Connor knew someone. We talked for a while longer, and I was really excited to tell Connor about Leah's suggestion.

4

THE START OF AN INVESTIGATION

Connor Jackson

I didn't go on a run that night because it wasn't in my training plan, but I went out of my way during my afternoon commute to drive past the building. Then I turned around and drove past it again, slowly. Finally, I just parked at the lot nearby. As I walked up the trail, I was aware of the many people around me, and I couldn't believe that I was really considering breaking into a building that I knew nothing about—not what it was, not even who owned it. I wished there was a bench near the building or some reason to stop near it. Also, in my scrubs, I didn't look like I needed to do some stretches or anything. But this time I was walking slowly instead of running and was looking at the building as I approached it, instead of out of the corner of my eye as I passed. Nothing had really changed since the day before, although the trail was dry and some sticks had been cleared. I was approaching the door at the same angle I had during my run. From this distance, I tried to inspect the ground within the fence and saw no tracks in the mud or evidence of animals. The fence itself had a gate with no lock, just one of those U handles that kept it closed. I got my phone out when I was right next to it and pretended to be sending a text, but I was actually taking a few pictures. I knew Katie and Pumpkin would want to see them. My resolve to find out what was inside the building grew a lot stronger on this second visit.

THE NEXT DAY, Katie was feeling the worse for wear. The drugs were taking their toll, as they were supposed to, but she was still enthusiastic. There were also more photos in her room and now balloons. No one had more visitors than Katie.

"Did you go on a run last night? Did you get into the building?" That was the first thing she said to me as I entered her room. Her voice was weak and she had her covers pulled all the way up.

"Well, good morning to you, too!" I responded. "No, I didn't run. Yesterday was a rest day, but I checked it out and took a few pictures for you." I pulled out my phone and found the pics. "Here."

She studied the photos intently as she got out of bed to start our normal morning vitals check. "Looks different from Google Maps."

"I thought we couldn't find it on there," I said, as she got on the scale, still holding my phone.

"We didn't look at the satellite images yesterday. I

looked again. And you can see it in the street view. You totally took a better picture! I couldn't see how tall the pole is. Wow!" I took her temporal temperature. The enthusiasm in her voice was high but her body slumped and she moved slowly.

Then I did the blood draw. Again, a pause in the conversation.

"You really did your homework on this thing, Katie!"

"Dude, I have nothing to do here other than watch daytime TV and wish I was with my kids." She paused, then whispered excitedly, "I also made some phone calls."

"You what?"

"Well, after I saw it was right beside the Park District's golf course, I thought I'd call and see what they knew." Katie found a blonde lock to curl around her fingers. "The District's Administration Office seemed pretty clueless about it and left me on hold a few times. I hung up eventually. Then I talked to the golf course manager, Leah something or other. I wrote it down over there. She said that she's been wondering about it, too. She's only been at the job for about six months and has been poking around. And she thinks it has to do with energy generation a long time ago, but she's not sure yet."

"Energy generation! Whoa!"

"She didn't say this, but I don't think it's high on her work to-do list since the golf course is hosting some 'golf outings' the next few weekends and closing down for the season soon." Katie put air quotes around "golf outings." I'd always found that a weird way to describe a golf fundraiser, too. You just call it a race when you're *running* for a charity!

"I can't believe you made with the phone calls and found out so much!" I said as I labeled her blood specimen and finished typing up my records. "Crazy that it's not on the Park District's radar. After being there last night, I decided that I really can't get into the building after work. It's too busy of a time. I'd have to go early in the morning or something." I paused and added, "I'm just not so sure about breaking into it. I don't think I'm the breaking-and-entering kind of guy." Just as I told Pumpkin.

"It's not like I can do it!" Katie scolded me. You've gotta get in there—for the both of us!"

"No, you can't do it," I agreed. "I'm thinking about it. Anyway, we need to get this next drug started, and I need to send your specimen to the lab. I'll be back in a few."

When I saw Katie again, her red-haired cousin with fluttery eyes had brought lunch and was chatting with her. I joined the conversation as I changed the IV bag. I could tell Katie was getting tired, so I didn't extend my visit. With five other patients that day, I didn't have time for long conversations.

As I was leaving for the night, I popped into Katie's room to check on her and she seemed to be napping, so I turned to leave.

"You don't have to be the breaking-and-entering kind of guy, Connor. Doing it once won't define you," Katie said, lifting her head, which pulled me back into the room.

"I'm going on a six-miler tonight with a faster pace in the middle. I'll run past our building and scope it out a bit more," I said, putting my hands in my jacket pockets and kicking at the sink cabinet near the door. "I guess you're right that doing something once doesn't define you."

"I'm not going to be a cancer patient forever, that's for sure. Being here for three weeks will change my life and make me healthier, but I will not let it define me. I think what we do at our lowest and at our highest and how we react to those things, how they change us—that defines us. Doing something once out of curiosity keeps life exciting, but doing something one time—that doesn't define you."

I nodded. People with cancer can be such sages sometimes. "Not going to let it define you. I hear you. See you on Monday, Katie. Rest easy." She closed her eyes, and I closed the door, not letting the latch click loudly.

———

I HAD a rare three days off in a row: Friday through Sunday. Usually, I work five weekdays one week and then four weekdays the next week with one weekend day. I switched with a coworker for an extra day shift the week before and so had a long weekend now.

It started raining on my way home. Rainy weather is perfect for a longer run, in my opinion, although I know many runners disagree. My lungs always feel good in wet weather. And the trail would be less crowded. The plop-plop of rain also makes for good thinking. I was pondering what Katie said about how actions do or do not define us. I really couldn't come up with an action that defined me other than how I treat the people surrounding me. I've always tried my hardest to be caring to my patients, loving to my nieces, friendly to my neighbors. And I run and play video games, but do those hobbies define me?

I had a plan to try out a new sweatband that just came in the mail from Amazon on these rainy six miles. Not a lady's headband that wraps around the back of her neck, but the kind basketball players wear across their foreheads. Like Lebron James. I bought it to keep my hair out of my eyes, but now I realized it would give me another excuse to pause while running by the building.

When I got home, I went over the postal mail while petting Pumpkin, who was sitting next to me on the counter. Then I changed for my run. I wore my older running shoes I don't mind getting muddy and donned my sweatband.

The building was about a half mile away on the paved loop trail. I was pretty soaked by the time I got there. The sweatband wasn't doing much for my hair since it was already stuck, wet, against my forehead. And I was right about the trail being less crowded. I hadn't met another person yet.

Seeing no one, I made no pretense of adjusting the sweatband or my shoes and squashed my way through the mud, past the huge tulip poplar, and right up to the chain-link fence. I had to dig the meat of my hand into the U handle before it moved upward. I wished I had brought some work gloves or maybe even a crowbar. The hinges were loud and squeaky as I pulled the gate toward me. I made my way around the corner of the building, stepping on poison ivy, prickly vines, and saplings. *Sorry, trees,* I thought. I really had to fight the vegetation, and by the time I was right in front of the door, my heart shouldn't have been beating as hard as it was from running. I had a lot of scratches on my left leg.

The doorknob was slick and didn't turn in my hand. I pushed at the wooden door, but it didn't move. I put my right eye up to the crack between the door and its jamb, trying to see inside before pushing farther. I could see a sliver of wooden floor and the brick walls. Maybe a wooden workbench along the far wall with some papers on it. I didn't see evidence of animals and barely any leaves or debris, but my view was small. I didn't want to get my phone out of my waterproof wrist strap to use the flashlight because of the rain.

Pushing harder on the door didn't open it. I tried to pull the door up so that it was straight in the doorjamb, but doing that didn't make it open either. I was getting nervous being inside the fence for so long. There is a road next to the trail, but it doesn't get much traffic, mostly just trail users. I gave up and thought I'd bring equipment next time. Katie would still be excited to hear anything I learned.

As I'd told Katie, this run was supposed to be an easy mile, then a faster pace for a few miles, and then easy again. I totally messed up the faster tempo pace in the middle of the run, but I thought the sacrifice was worth the extra information. I ran an extra half mile to make up for it. And pushing on a door is not the same as breaking and entering, right?

5

THE FOOD ORDER

Katie Brandt

By day four, I was over the hospital food. I'd had their sad little salad three times, their mushy french fries twice, and never wanted the baked chicken again. The french bread pizza tasted nothing like pizza I'd had before: soggy crust, super-sweet sauce, and not enough cheese. None of it was great, although it sounded appealing on the first day. Having worked in another hospital as a surgical tech, I had a hunch there was food not on my menu that I might be able to work my way into.

This hospital had a number to call to order your meals. You couldn't order ahead, so I placed three calls a day. I called at about four, before dinner, and Renee answered, asking for my order. I greeted her, using her name, my room number, and my own name.

"Can they send me up an alternate menu, please, Renee? Can I try the employee or guest menu, perhaps?"

"Patients are supposed to order from the patient menu. You need a doctor's orders to change menus. Sorry."

"Are you a cook, Renee?" I didn't want to offend her and reminded myself that Renee might have been having a hard day. I wouldn't want her job taking food orders on the phone all day!

"No, I am not," she reported, very to the point.

"Well, I'm not going to lie, but the patient menu is pretty mushy and tasteless. It's not like I need to be on a low-sodium or fluid diet. Have you had any of the food?"

"No, I have not." Again, short, but not mad. I decided to play the celebrity card that I somehow held.

"I'm going to be here for three weeks, Renee. I know you guys have a larger variety of food in the cafeteria. I'm a cancer survivor. I was pregnant with high-risk twins while having my chemo treatments. You might have seen me and my family on the news or even in your hospital newsletter," I said as quickly as I could. This high-risk twin thing was kind of subjective, but the news people had really latched on to it. It was always really weird to see myself on TV, in the newspaper, or in some other media. You'd think all the press would have amounted to something, but so far, it hadn't even gotten me good food in the hospital. "I'd just really appreciate your help to get something tasty today!" I concluded.

"Oh! You're that lady? You've really had it rough," Renee told me, her tone changing drastically.

"So, can I order something that's not on the patient menu?"

"What you need to do is go to our cafeteria website

and see what we're offering today. You tell me what you want, and I'll have it sent up to you," she said.

"You're a lifesaver, Renee. This food would have killed me! I'll call you back in a few minutes."

As my food was being prepared, I thought about the food I'd ordered at this same hospital when I was having chemo, which led me down the rabbit hole of thinking about when Travis and I first were told we were having twins and all that followed.

I'll never forget Travis's smile when the ultrasound tech told us there were two babies. He was holding my hand and smiling bigger than I've ever seen him smile. I mean, huge. Nothing like this when he proposed or when he caught a thirty-pound grouper off the coast of Florida.

And sure, I wanted to be pregnant. We wanted another kid, but when that tech told us there were two in my tummy in early September the year before, I did not smile like my crazy husband. My mind had raced. How in the world I would handle two more babies plus our sweet toddler PJ. This felt like madness. But, man, Travis was smiling for both of us, and I couldn't help but smile with him. We were having twins!

We made quiet announcements to our inner circle at PJ's second birthday party in late September, and our families were ecstatic. It was a really happy few weeks.

But it wasn't a good pregnancy. I was always tired. I mean, always tired. Headaches and backaches plagued me, and I was coughing. In October, when they took the twelve-week blood test, there was a lot of concern. None of the doctors in my OB-GYN practice had seen results like this, so they went searching medical journals. That took some time, and I was feeling worse and, honestly, terrified.

One week, I lost seven pounds.

Let that settle in a minute. I lost seven pounds in one week. When I was pregnant. I couldn't have done that if I'd worked out every day and counted calories. So needless to say, I was freaking out. I was really worried about my babies, and no one could tell me what was happening yet.

A few weeks later, my obstetrician's office had an answer. The blood test result that was most concerning had been found in only ten pregnant women in the world. A sample size of ten isn't a good test of anything, but all these ladies had something in common.

They all had cancer.

The problem was, we didn't know where the cancer was yet. So I had more blood tests, an MRI, a CAT scan, a bone biopsy. These aren't fun tests for anyone, let alone a really uncomfortable, tired, pregnant lady trying her best to run around after a two-year-old. It took time to schedule those tests and then get the results. I felt like my mom and I were constantly at medical facilities.

I'm a big worrier, so being told I had cancer was itself toxic to me. I think some headaches I experienced were stress related.

I was working part-time as a surgical tech in a nearby hospital's operating room. I spent most of my time at home caring for PJ, but my worsening condition made it hard to do anything well. Almost every day, my mom, my sister, my cousin, my mother-in-law, or someone else was at my house or picking up my kiddo. We were so lucky to have such a village of caring people around us. Within a month, my employer put me on disability and I no longer had to work. I wanted to be upset about not being able to do a job I loved, but I was so tired and not doing it to the best of my ability.

Finally, they did a chest X-ray, compared it to a past X-ray, and saw nodes that shouldn't be there. Yes, I had been a smoker years ago. Was this lung cancer? More tests showed prominent lymph nodes in my armpits and neck. They did a biopsy, and we waited.

One of my sisters, Karissa, was getting married in the middle of this crazy time. That always happens, doesn't it? You're busy when insane things are going on around you. It was a happy distraction. By mid-November, I wasn't able to drive anymore. I was too tired and weak. On the way to the wedding reception, I was looking up test results on my phone when I saw it in black and white: I had lymphoma. I didn't tell any of my family until after the wedding, but no one was surprised.

And another test the following week narrowed it further to Hodgkin's lymphoma. Naming this enemy that was taking away all my energy felt good. We knew who the fight was against now. I was going to kick its butt—right after a nap.

Usually, Hodgkin's is treatable, winnable. But it's very unusual to be pregnant and have any cancer, let alone be pregnant with twins. So we had an altered treatment plan. Most patients have both radiation and several chemo drugs. I would be getting reduced amounts of easier chemo drugs—starting the following week—and nothing else. Again, I am a worrier, and really had to be convinced that my babies would be okay after this treatment.

I had eleven rounds of chemo throughout the next few months, often every other week. I have a finicky immune system to start with and was allergic to some of what they wanted to use.

My mom always came with me for chemo treatments. We got to know the nurses on the cancer treatment floor well. My first few rounds, I sat in the big, white reclining chairs that all the other cancer patients used. But when I was further along in my pregnancy, they wanted to monitor the girls more closely, and I got a private room.

I'll never forget the time that my care team reacted faster than I did to my allergies. I was in my room. My mom was there, and so was my cousin Rachel. I had been there an hour for the pre-meds before the actual chemo drugs started, both administered via a port in my neck where they could just insert a needle, instead of sticking me in the arm with an IV every other week.

My mom and cousin sat in smaller, less plush chairs next to my big recliner. We had settled in, having already exchanged plenty of chitchat, and were reading books and magazines. I had my legs up and was covered in a blanket because I was always chilly back then. The chemo drugs started, and mom left the room to use the bathroom. Her return started some conversation, and I said, "I'm feeling itchy," without really giving it much notice or thought.

"Itchy?" Rachel asked. "That doesn't seem right."

"You might be a little flushed, honey," my mom said, stepping closer to look at my face.

"Yeah. I don't know," I said, feeling a bit embarrassed.

I opened up my book again, trying to shrug it off. Mom and Rachel looked at each other, but I didn't make eye contact, focusing on the words on the page. But within the next minute, my tongue felt weird, too thick and tingly.

"Thactually. Thi don' feel so goo," I said, trying to tell them about my tongue, but it wasn't responding the way I wanted it to.

Nodding decisively, my mom said, "I'll get the nurse," while Rachel stood up and pushed the call button.

My mom couldn't have even reached the nurse's station before ten nurses were by my side. Ten! Plus my oncologist. Someone whisked away my blanket and book. A blonde nurse in plaid scrubs replaced my drug bag with a different one in seconds. Another nurse with long braids put an oxygen mask over my mouth and nose with exacting precision, while a male nurse with a goatee turned me on my side. Someone I couldn't see poked a needle into my right thigh. The doctor looked into my eyes with his small flashlight. My mom reappeared in the doorway, and my cousin stood by the wall to be out of their way. I looked at both of them, making eye contact, and I just started giggling. This was madness!

I ended up having hives all over my arms, neck, and face. My flushed face was the start of the hives. They took a few hours to subside. My tongue went back to normal quickly. They had given me strong doses of baby-safe Benadryl that helped calm my body.

Once the allergic reaction had subsided, the doc came back. "Well, I guess we'll never be using that chemo drug again, will we?" He chuckled, but his tone was one of concern. "We've made notes in your chart and are always going to make sure we have a crash cart of allergy response supplies nearby for you. I don't want to take any chances of that happening again. We need to keep you and your little ones safe." My mom and I nodded. "We were lucky that the team was so quick and worked so well together." He smiled at that last part, with pride in his voice.

6

THE BIRTHDAY PARTY

Connor Jackson

On Fridays, I have a standing "running meeting" with my buddy, Eduardo, from my old job. We change up the time depending on our shifts, and he worked until four that day. He's slower than me, and it really worked out that my plan called for three easy miles. Ed's a bodybuilder and a phenomenal nurse. Both of his parents are from the Dominican Republic, but he was born in America. He has a little boy named Alvin who's three years old. As a bodybuilder, Ed is at the gym four days a week and wanted to incorporate more cardio into his workout regime, so he started running with me a bit. Before Alvin was born, I tried some weight lifting with Eduardo and it was just sad. I hated it. But he enjoyed running with me, so we kept it up and had a good reason to see each other every week.

This Friday, we ran around his neighborhood before his shift. Sometimes we meet at a Park District trail, the

Buckeye Trail on the other side of town, or run at the field house at the YMCA, where he's a member in the colder months.

After the run, I dug into my well-worn copy of the *Complete Sherlock Holmes*. I had a hankering to reread the *Hound of the Baskervilles* and finished it that morning.

That night, I got Indian takeout from my favorite restaurant, Saffron and Naan, and watched a movie as I wrapped some presents. I also poked around on my computer, looking up the golf course and the map Katie had seen. When I searched for old energy-generation buildings, I found nothing in this area. I stared at the pictures on my phone of the pole attached to the building and searched for what could be at the end of a tall pole. Maybe it had something to do with wind energy. I found out that you study wind velocity for wind energy generation with an anemometer. Maybe that's what the pole was, but old and no longer used? I ended up emailing some wind power nonprofit groups to ask if the attached photo was an anemometer.

———

I HAD BEEN LOOKING FORWARD to Saturday for a long time—except for the cross-training I had to do. At the rec center, I put in my forty minutes on the elliptical. No matter what I chose to do on cross-training days, I always struggled to stave off boredom. I thought next time I'd try swimming again.

This particular Saturday was my niece Chloe's fifth

birthday party. I call her Clover. Her older sister, June, is one of my very favorite people. Not that I play favorites. It's just that Juney has more to say and is into Harry Potter and building Lego, which are more exciting to me than the Disney princess stuff Clover likes the most. Being an uncle definitely defines me.

Juney and Clover are my brother Levi's kids. He's four years older and lives about twenty minutes away. We both work at the same hospital but never run into each other. He's a certified registered nurse anesthetist (CRNA), so he makes bigger bucks but works more hours. His operating room is on the other side of the campus. His wife, Erin, also works at the hospital in the outpatient recovery room, so they get to see each other when they're both working. She works part-time to be with the girls more. Our mom was also an RN before she retired; maybe we've all got that medical gene. Well, Dad is still the principal at our elementary school, so maybe I can't quite say that.

Levi and I have always been close even though we were four years apart in school. We've got the normal competitive brother relationship, too. Although we weren't in high school or college together, we attended the same state college about an hour's drive from our hometown and joined the same fraternity. Levi got a basketball scholarship to college. He's three inches taller than me. I kind of always knew I couldn't keep up with him athletically, although I ran track and competed well. I was the brain of the family and got academic scholarships that he did not. Back then, I had my eyes set on being a doctor.

After cleaning up, I headed to Levi's. As I was

walking up the brick driveway to enter their house through the garage, I could hear Erin yelling: "Uncle Connor is here, girls!" Then cheering. I'm a popular guy in this house. I was early on purpose.

I had five wrapped packages with me. Chloe was turning five, and I had started this birthday number of gifts too long ago to not carry on the tradition. And I go all out on the wrapping for these girls. Not so much for anyone else. I got her Disney Lego set because I knew Clover had wanted to play with Juney's Lego. An Elsa dress-up outfit *with heels* (wrapped separately), candy I know Levi isn't a fan of, and a pack of one thousand glow-in-the-dark stars. You know: the good stuff.

As I entered the house, I got tackled by their brown mutt, Howie, and then Clover and Juney. Hugs and kisses all around, jumping and squealing about the gifts. I almost dropped the bottle of Erin's favorite pinot I'd brought. That's the way to make an entrance. I kissed Erin on the cheek and did the traditional bro-hug with Levi. I was with my people.

They'd decked the place out with princess decor. Erin's family makes a big deal about birthdays. They'd have at least thirty people for the party: neighbors, kid friends, grown-up friends, and our family. They set a bounce house up in the backyard, and a croquet course in the side yard. I helped put beer and sodas in a cooler of ice on the deck and set up some folding tables on the lawn.

My parents' arrival produced a similar jumping-and-hugging reaction from the girls, although I liked to tell myself that they got more excited about their cool uncle.

The girls called my parents "Gramp" and "Gram Gram," and the adoration went both ways. I didn't squeal and jump myself, but my parents held a lot of weight in my life and I was glad to see them too. After they arrived, but before anyone else did, I pulled Juney aside in the dining room.

"How's my favorite almost eight-year-old?"

"School starts the week after next. I'm going to miss the summer," she said, pouting.

"Yeah, summer breaks always go way too fast. We need to plan another sleepover soon. Maybe the first weekend you're in school, so you have something to look forward to?"

Of the three bedrooms in my condo, one is mine, of course. One is an "office," which just means it has a desk, a scratching post for Pumpkin, a file cabinet, and a bunch of boxes of junk. I always end up with my laptop on the couch and don't use the desk at all. My guest room holds a bunk bed with a queen-size mattress on the bottom and a twin on top. The bunk beds have pink comforters and sheets. I got them on clearance, but they get used the most because my nieces are my most frequent guests. I also have a Lego Friends poster on the wall and totally own the Disney Elsa and Anna poster next to it. For other guests, like my college buddies, I throw on gray sheets and the afghan from Stephanie. I don't make them sleep in pink. But I leave the posters. They know why I've got girly kid posters in my guest room.

Juney liked the idea of a sleepover. When they're staying, I take them to the playground in my development and we walk to get ice cream when it's warm. We usually get pizza, watch a movie, and eat popcorn popped on the stove. They get excited about that. It's all about the food.

"I picked up a new minifig bag," I told her patting my chest and legs, acting like I was looking for it in pockets that weren't on my clothes like the ridiculous grown-up that I am. Minifigs are the "minifigure" people in Lego sets. The company sells some individually in mystery bags that don't tell you which character they contain, changing the theme every few months. These blind bags are a great way to sell tons of them because kids always want a specific minifig, and you just never know which one you'll get. Juney really wanted the Hermione figure.

"You got another one in the Harry Potter series?" She was flapping her hands and rocking on the balls of her feet. I love how excited kids get!

"Yeah, the big-box store is really hiding them nowadays. I hope we can keep finding them." I finally found it: right in the back pocket of my jeans, the last place anyone would look. She retrieved a pair of kid-size scissors from the kitchen. Those minifig bags are hard for anyone to open. I bought five bags last time I was at the store so I would be set for the next few times I saw her.

"Aw, man. Another Dobby," she announced, crestfallen. Dobby was a minor but really popular character in the Harry Potter books. Unfortunately, he was not her favorite.

"You know, why don't we put him in your room at my house? I don't have any minifigs there yet."

"That sounds good. Dobby *is* pretty cool, though. I like how he hid the sock in the book."

"Sock in the book! Yep! Sneaky Harry Potter!" I

agreed. In the magical world, sometimes all you need is a hidden sock in a book to set a guy free from slavery."

She put the little guy together, and we made our way outside. Clover was already sweaty from jumping in the bounce house. I said hello to some more family members who had arrived. My Uncle Dave and Aunt Peg couldn't agree whether my longer hair looked good or not.

I was sitting at a folding table talking with one of Levi's coworkers when I saw someone I had never seen at one of these parties before. She was on the deck talking to Erin and had long brown hair pulled into a ponytail and bangs. First impression: she was hot. I excused myself and headed for the grill on the patio. Levi was piling freshly grilled brats onto a tray, and I asked him who she was.

"Oh, you know Erin. She invites everyone she knows to our parties. That's Leah. She's new to Erin's spinning class. I guess their bikes are next to each other and they've really hit it off," he said.

"So . . . ah . . ."

"Let me introduce you, little bro." He loves to call me that. He kind of shoved me toward the deck with his arm around my shoulders, balancing the brats like an expert and grinning from ear to ear.

"Hey, Leah. Did you get a beer? My brother, Connor, also brought some wine if you're interested in that. It's inside. I've got brats too!" Levi said, holding his tray aloft and dripping with charisma.

"Hey, Levi! Hi, Connor. Nice to meet you. Yeah, some wine and a brat both sound great," she said, her eyes darting from me to my brother.

"It's in here," I told her awkwardly, leading the way

into the kitchen through the sliding glass door. I felt like I was marching in a parade and also felt my middle school awkwardness rising again.

"You guys have a beautiful house. I'm honored to be invited to the big five birthday party!" Leah said to Levi with a smile.

"We like to celebrate everything with everyone! I'm glad you're here," Levi told her as I got the wineglasses out of the cabinet and fumbled through the utensils drawer for the corkscrew. Levi put his tray of brats on the counter next to a Crock-Pot of baked beans.

"Thanks," she said, but Levi didn't let her say anything else. The charismatic guy act dropped, and he rushed to tell her: "Help yourself to any of the food. Here are the plates. Gotta get back out there and man the grill." He booked it out the door before either of us could respond. She blinked after him.

"So, do you like pinot? This is Erin's favorite wine-maker," I said, unsure that "winemaker" was the right term to use at all. She turned and smiled at me, obviously a bit taken aback by Levi's quick exit and turn in mood.

"Well, if it's Erin's favorite, I should try it!" she said. I uncorked the bottle and poured her a glass. I had left my beer outside, so I took another beer out of the fridge. This was Levi's stash, not the cheaper stuff from the coolers. I told her so much.

We talked about alcohol for a few minutes and I found my calm again, losing the preteen awkwardness that always bubbles to the surface when I'm around any pretty lady. She told me how she'd met Erin in spinning class, and we crept into the empty formal living room in front of the house. I told her about my half-marathon coming up and that I had never been to a spinning class. I was being funny, maybe even cool.

"Yeah, so I'm in the medical field too, like Erin and Levi. I'm a nurse on the stem cell replacement ward at the hospital. We're all at the same place every day but never see each other." I thought we were hitting it off pretty well until she hit me with a bit of a bomb.

"Stem cell replacement? That's serious stuff! I can't imagine the people you see every day! I just deal with golfers. They can be serious about the sport, but no one's life is at stake. I manage the Peregrine Falcon Golf Club. I just moved back to the area this year to be closer to my family."

The Peregrine Falcon Golf Club was the golf course right next to my trail; this Leah had to be the same Leah that Katie had talked to this week! I didn't recover well. "You . . . ah . . . You manage the golf course?" I panicked and wanted to blurt out that she had talked to my patient but didn't know what to do. Instead, I started crazily scratching the poison ivy on my leg from the expedition to the building. It really itched suddenly, and somehow I felt like this let me stall. For a full minute.

"I do. Are you a golfer, Connor?" she asked after I said nothing for so long. She was leaning down to look at my leg.

"I got poison ivy the other day. Do you deal with a lot of that on the golf course?" I knew that didn't sound cool. I didn't even answer her question. I'm not a golfer.

"Oh, well, I'm not on the grounds crew or anything. I'm not into the turf management side of things. I manage the events and employees, mostly. But yeah, I've seen some ivy on the wooded edges of the course."

Thankfully, at this point Erin called everyone to the deck to watch Chloe blow out the candles on her cake. I downed my beer and grabbed another cheap one from the deck cooler. We all sang loudly for Clover, who soaked it all up. She loved to be the center of attention.

I found Juney and chased her around the yard through the croquet hoops until Levi gave us plates of cake and ice cream. We were some of the last to get our desserts. I sat with her under a tree as we ate. I saw Leah at a folding table across the lawn and knew I couldn't leave our conversation hanging for so long.

"Now, don't jump on the bounce house for at least, like, fifteen minutes after eating, okay?" I warned Juney after we were done. I doubted this uncle-instruction after I said it. Maybe it really should have been an hour or something? "I'll take our plates in," I said, getting up.

Instead of heading to the house, I walked up to Leah, who was talking to another friend of Erin's. I couldn't remember her name, but I'd met her plenty of times. "Want me to take your plates in the house?" I asked, totally interrupting their conversation and grabbing plates from around the table. I'd blame the rudeness on the beer if necessary.

"Oh, hi, Connor!" What's-her-name said. "Yeah, thanks, we were just finishing up. Do you know if Chloe will open her presents during the party or not? I forget if Levi and Erin wait until after guests leave to do the presents."

"Yeah, they do usually wait," I said. I still don't get

this: I guess it's to make people not feel bad if they gave a cheaper gift than other people? I'd be staying late to watch her open *my* awesome gifts. I needed to see that little girl in her first heels! While stacking up all the plates, I made eye contact with Leah. "Do you think you could help me, Leah?" I asked, pretending I couldn't handle all the plates in the many stacks I had made.

"Oh sure," she said, taking three plates. Only three. She knew what was going on.

After we were out of earshot of that other lady, I finally found my nerve. "So, about this golf course. I wanted to talk to you more about it. Sorry, I got kind of weird about poison ivy."

"Yeah. What's up?"

"Let's go on the porch," I said.

7

THE PORCH

Connor Jackson

After loading the plates into the sink, I led Leah to the front porch. This seemed extra private since no one was even in the front room. We settled into the red Adirondack chairs, and I jumped in.

"I'll just get straight to it," I said. "You got a phone call this week about a little building on the edge of the golf course, right? The brick building with the tall pole?"

"I did. How do you know?" she asked, looking at me sideways.

"I know the person who called you, and I told her about the building. She hasn't actually seen it for herself. She's a patient of mine, Katie."

"Oh. Your patient?" Leah leaned back in her chair and crossed her arms. I didn't feel like this was going so well.

"I run past the building a few times a week. It's on a trail behind my condo. That storm a few nights ago seems to have knocked the door free and now it's open a bit. Like the door is hanging off the hinges. I admit that I've gotten obsessed with the building since the door broke. It's really weird to meet you this same week." I took a deep breath and waited for her response. She took a deep breath at the same time.

"Yeah, that is really weird," she agreed.

"So. Have you seen the door?" I asked quickly. "You told her you thought the building had something to do with power generation."

"No, I haven't been over to that corner of the course lately. Haven't seen the door," she said thoughtfully and paused. She seemed to be deciding if I was a mental patient or not. "You had a patient call me?"

"Oh, I really didn't tell her to, trust me!"

"But she did!" she accused me, eyes wide, leaning forward.

"Katie is a real go-getter. She's stuck in the hospital, and this really caught her attention because she's so bored. She found out more about it than I did! She'll be thrilled when I tell her I met you without meaning to."

"It *is* such a coincidence. So you didn't tell her to call me?" I shook my head no, and she seemed to believe me and uncrossed her arms. "Well, I had to look in our archives at the Park District admin building. I don't really get there very often, either. The building is only on some of our older maps."

"On some of your older maps! What did the maps say about it?"

"The golf course was donated to the Park District twelve years ago. From what I understand, the former owners neglected it, and we're still doing renovations while keeping the surrounding nature intact and thriving. Staying 'green' and all that. We're the Park District first. And there's a lot to do on three hundred and fifty acres, right?"

"Makes sense," I said. "I didn't realize the Park District hasn't owned it for that long. Was the building donated with the golf course?"

"Yeah, the building is on the same tract of land. The thing is, the building is not on any current golf course maps and not on our aerial maps because of all the surrounding trees." She leaned forward, and continued conspiratorially. "I was at the admin office a couple of weeks ago for a staff meeting and nosed around in our old files. The property itself has been nothing but a golf course, practically a nature preserve. There were farms around it in the 1800s, and I think that's when that little building was built. It was on those really old maps way before it was a golf course," she explained, her face lit up, excited.

"Wow! It's that old? But it's not on current maps?"

"Not on current maps of the *golf course*, but it *is* on maps of the entire park system."

"That's an interesting distinction. I wonder why," I said.

"Right, I don't know. I'm not sure who to ask." Leah was picking at her thumbnail and looking across the street, off into the distance. "I should get over there and see the broken door now. It's all just so interesting!"

I looked across the street, too. She really seemed into finding out more about the building, searching old maps and all. But could I ask her to break into it with me? I changed the subject.

"I really haven't been golfing since I was in high school. I think I'd like to try again."

A smile cracked her face as she focused her attention back on me. "Well, as it happens, I teach lessons. Unless you want to try the course on your own with no practice?"

"Well, what do you suggest?" I asked, leaning forward with a big grin.

"Seems to me you probably need some practice," she said in a joking voice.

"Let's set up a time," I said, and she raised her eyebrows. "I'm serious. Do you give lessons at, like, 4:30 any day this week?"

"I'd have to check my schedule, but I probably have an opening."

"So, should I call the golf course? Or, ah . . . should I get your number?" Levi would have been more suave, but that was all I could come up with.

"Yeah, let's exchange numbers," Leah agreed, standing up and getting out her phone. I took mine out of my pocket as I stood up and found the new contacts section.

"I'm not done talking about the building," I told her after we put away our phones again.

"Me neither," she said with a smile. She had a really pretty smile, such straight, white teeth.

I stayed until it was the girls' bedtime that night. Clover loved every single present she got and wore the heels until bath time. It was a great day.

8

THE ELEVEN-MILE RUN

Connor Jackson

My race was exactly three weeks away, and I doubted I was ready at all. Eleven miles sounded really far. It felt really far when I was running it. My knees and feet were feeling it at the end, and I was going slower than I wanted to. I forgot the headband on my last run and remembered it for this one. It just made me more sweaty. Either my hair was bouncing up and down on top of it or was even more plastered against my forehead under it.

As I passed the building this time, I just slowed down. No need to break in yet. I just stared it down, mentally saying hello.

I've always done my best thinking while running. I rarely listen to music unless I'm on a treadmill. During this run, I was thinking again about Katie. She and I were both doing something physically hard on purpose. Of course, all my patients do, but Katie was top of mind. I was running more than I usually do, putting my body to the test, for a greater athletic achievement. Katie was hurting her immune system for overall better health. It was a cool parallel. Thinking about Katie also made me think about our conversation about what defined me. I decided that being a caretaker, a nurse, defined me the most. I realized I hadn't thought about why in a long time.

My desire to be a doctor in high school changed during my last few years of college, after I met Clayton in the obligatory psychology class that every student who goes to college is required to take. I hated it but, as always, strove to do well. Clay was an English major with a history minor, hoping to get his PhD to teach history at the college level. He was a funny guy who made me laugh out loud in class, and we hit it off right away. He had a crazy memory and bleached blond hair and was also a runner. We ended up running a lot together. He joined my fraternity, too, so we saw each other often. But in the second semester of sophomore year, he got sick, and no one knew why. He just kept losing weight, having back-aches, and sleeping all the time, but never got better. Over the summer, he was diagnosed with pancreatic cancer. That type of cancer is hard to beat. Thankfully, our hospital—where I work now—was near enough to the college that he could get chemo there because he refused to take any time off of school. I ended up staying with him frequently, studying in his room at the hospital because he was so sick. And I saw the care he was given. I saw that the doctors came in once a day, twice, maybe. But the nurses were the people on the ground who helped the patients feel better, who provided the daily care. The doctors made the decisions, and the nurses carried them out.

Clay died before Thanksgiving break. It was a crazy low time in my life. Losing anyone is hard, but losing your best friend when you are young yourself is insanity. I don't know how I took any finals, let alone passed them. That Christmas break is still a blur of grief and running at the YMCA. As you'd expect, my parents and Levi carried me through. My adviser helped me switch classes and take a really easy course load the next semester. Then I enrolled in the nursing program the following year. I had to take a lot more classes and stay on an extra year to get it all in. I was a dedicated student and did what I needed to. I've had such a clarity of career choices since losing Clay. And so this loss, this friendship, has defined pretty much my entire life. Caring for sick people defines who I am.

————

AFTER THE ELEVEN miles had been checked off on my training plan, I iced my feet, downed ibuprofen, and drank some electrolytes. Pumpkin liked it when I iced my feet. He pushed the ice around the bowl and splashed water onto the floor.

This wasn't the first time I'd trained for a half-marathon. I did one two years ago with Ed. The entire race happened during a downpour, and it was one of those odd forty-five-degree September mornings with frost. A downpour is different from the relaxing rain I like to run in. I wasn't quite ready—I hadn't done my last long run and had skipped most cross-training days. Ed did horribly, too, and he swore off running longer distances after it. Between my lackadaisical training and the weather, I finished at 2:10:36. I was really unhappy with my time and knew that I needed to run another one to be satisfied. My primary goal was to finish the race in under two hours this time around, but I'd really like to be well under two.

My normal runs were about five miles, or just over, on the trail loop that led to my patio. I really enjoyed the seven-mile route along the stream on the Buckeye Trail nearby, but I needed to drive to get to it, so I only went there a few times a month unless I was training for a race. Call it laziness. I do a few 5Ks and 10Ks every summer, usually doing well in my age group. So a half-marathon, at 13.1 miles, was well beyond my normal, a good challenge. And it was proving to be. The mental challenge of any race was the hardest part, but I trusted my training plan and hadn't messed up yet. And I was being kind to my feet: no flip-flops that summer. When I wasn't running, I wore work shoes or running shoes that had been worn out but were still intact.

All day, I really, really wanted to text or call Leah. I wanted to know where she lived before she moved here and what got her into golf course management. I also realized that she didn't tell me why she thought the building had anything to do with making electricity by the end of our conversation. Instead of calling her, I settled on calling the golf course to set up a lesson with her for Tuesday. I'd text her on Monday, I decided. That's the cool guy rule. Wait a day before contact. Did she know I was interested in her romantically? Was that obvious at all? Did she think I was only talking to her to learn about the building? Or golf lessons?

9

THE BUILDING AND KATIE

Connor Jackson

On Monday, I was back at work and sore from the long run. It was an "either rest or cross-train" day. I decided to just do some stretches, sit-ups, and push-ups in the morning and call it a suitable medium. I convinced myself this wasn't cheating.

I was really excited to talk to Katie but knew that her treatments must have left her in a bad place since I had seen her three days ago. My sore legs were nothing in comparison. That's one good thing about seeing cancer patients every day. It keeps you grounded, knowing that what you have going on isn't as bad as what they have going on. It makes everyone who works there appreciate being healthy, that's for sure.

When I looked in on her a few minutes after seven, she was sleeping but didn't look comfortable; her arms rested on top of the covers, and her head was propped up on a bunch of pink pillows. Her last vital readings from the night before were fine, and her white blood cells and ANC had tanked, which was what we wanted to see. I glimpsed more encouragement on the windows: a few new homemade cards lined the windowsill, and a beaded blue heart was taped to the wall with the pictures.

When I entered her room later, it was eight thirty and Katie was sitting up and ordering breakfast. "Katie! Tell me how you're feeling," I burst out, trying not to tell her everything that had happened over the weekend right away.

"Oh, man, I'm worn down. I'm feeling really tired but not getting good sleep."

"Are you feeling sick to your stomach? Headaches? I'll help you stand up." I gently pulled the covers back to help her up.

"Yes, and yes but I felt better before. They gave me some Onadostrone for nausea in the middle of the night, but it seems that it wore off. My body aches; my head aches." I took her hands and pulled her out of the bed.

She stood on the scale and then collapsed back into her soft quilt. I took some vitals.

"Yeah, I see your meds from last night in the chart," I finally said, looking at my laptop. "I can go get some more. You're about due. Maybe we can do a bigger dose, and that will help. I think the doc will be in about 9:30 this morning. We'll wait to start any other treatments until after we get his consult. Your vitals haven't changed since last time. That's good."

I checked on the patient next door, who was finishing his treatments and would probably be discharged the next day. I checked out Katie's meds and headed back to her room.

"Got the goods here!" I said. This larger dose was a tablet that went under the tongue, where it would be quickly absorbed into her body. "So, I had a big weekend. I know you didn't go anywhere, but you will not believe who I met." I don't know how I'd held in the news this long.

"Connor, don't make me guess. But tell me all the stories. I need good news here." Her enthusiasm showed only in the words, her excited body language long gone.

"Remember the golf course manager you called last week? Leah something, you said?" Katie sat up just a little straighter. She knew where I was going. "She was at my niece's birthday party!"

"Shut up!" Katie almost yelled. Her eyes were wide, but her body just wasn't doing anything else. I knew she wanted to. A low white blood cell count could do that to you. Her weakness was real.

"No kidding! She's a friend of my sister-in-law. How crazy is that?"

"Tell me you asked her about the building."

"I did! She told me she has been doing some digging and wondering about it like we have. She found it on some old maps at the Park District HQ. It was built in the early 1800s before there was a golf course there, just farms."

"That's a lot older than I thought. What else did she say?" Katie had slid back onto her pillows and covered her arms with the pink quilt, cocooning herself.

"It used to be kind of a nature preserve. The golf course hasn't been owned by the district for that long."

"Okay. But she told me she thought it had to do with making electricity. What about that?" Katie asked slowly.

"We didn't get that far, actually. That's all she really said." My news about meeting a pretty girl didn't seem as exciting as I had hoped. I didn't have as much info on the building as I had about meeting Leah. "I'm going to see her again on Tuesday, though, tomorrow. I'll ask her then."

"You're seeing her again? Like on a date? Connor, you asked her on a date?"

"She's giving me a golf lesson." I felt defensive but knew I didn't need to be. Katie was cool. "She's cute. It's not really a date. But maybe it is."

"Tuesday feels too far away. I'm barely going to make it through today."

"Your meds will kick in soon. I'll be back when the doctor is here." She closed her eyes without saying anything else, and I padded out.

———

SEEING AS IT WAS MONDAY, and into the cool guy response time, I texted Leah midmorning:

Connor: Hey, Leah, it's Connor, Erin's bro in law. I'll see you tomorrow for our golf lesson!

Her response was almost instant.

Leah: Connor! I'm excited to convert you into a golfer!

Connor: I think I need to convert you into a runner! See you then!

All day I was trying to work up the nerve to ask her to dinner after the lesson but was too busy, and, well, the nerve never showed up.

10

THE LAST CHEMO

Katie Brandt

E ach time I received a chemo treatment, it felt risky. My care team was always nervous that I'd have an allergic reaction, as I had before. Yet my very last dose of chemo was anticlimactic. It felt like such a milestone, such a goal that I was reaching for. It was on my calendar long before I was admitted into the hospital—and on the calendars of my people, too. But that last dose with Connor just felt too normal.

"We have to make this a big deal," I told Connor, when he came in carrying the IV bag.

"Well, it is a big deal, Katie! Last chemo of your life!" he said, always the enthusiastic optimist.

"I sure hope so," I said, feeling antsy and unsure—and so tired. He stood next to my bed, waiting for my celebratory instructions. I looked at him and then the bag for a long time. Then I looked out the window.

"What should we do?" he asked, when I didn't move and he was just standing there holding the drug bag.

"At least let's take a picture," I said. I opened the camera app and took a selfie of us and the syringe, ready to go into my neck port.

"Seems like not enough for you," he said as we looked at the photo. "Should I have frowned or something instead of a smile? Maybe we could take another with mean faces? Like we're mad?" Connor acting mad made me want to laugh.

"No, it was fine," I said, cracking a smile. He smiled back.

"Okay, what about this? What if we say 'say a few words'—like you do at a funeral? Like we're laying cancer to rest?"

"Wow! Did you just think of that? Have you done this for all the patients?" I teased him, though I hardly had the energy. Even so, Connor was always so easy to tease.

"Well, no. We don't have to do it if you don't want," he said, trying to shrug it off and act as if his feelings weren't hurt.

"No! It's great. Let's say a few words." I paused, thinking. Putting cancer to rest was a good idea. "So long, cancer. You suck, and I won't miss you at all."

"You've taken up too much of Katie's life and attention, cancer. Good riddance," Connor said, with his fake mean face.

"Everyone is happy to see you go," I added.

"We've worked hard to make sure you're dead. Get out of here!"

"You've lived a worthless life that caused too much pain. Too much pain for my babies and my family," I told cancer, tears welling in my eyes that I didn't expect. I had spent too much of my kids' young lives away from them, beating back cancer.

"And today, we lay you to rest," Connor said in a final, somber way to close up our funeral.

"I can't wait to see you go and be done. Rest in . . . in no peace." I nodded, wiped my eyes, and adjusted the collar on my shirt again. "Let's do it."

And Connor injected the drugs, the IV drip started, and it was over in about two hours, just like the rest of them. My last chemo injection was done without a parade, without pomp or a party, just a sad little funeral.

As I've mentioned, I often felt really amped up and not really able to rest or sleep for hours following chemo drugs, no matter how tired I was. After the injection, I ordered my lunch from Renee and got up to walk the halls with my IV on wheels. I talked to my mom as I walked. She was watching the girls, and I heard their sweet, wordless voices. One day I'd know them apart on the phone, but today their babbles still sounded the same. I cried after we got off the phone because I missed Travis, those little girls, and my sweet little man so much. I hated being stuck in this hospital.

When I got back to my room, I sat in the chair by the window that most of my visitors sat in. I decided I enjoyed addressing cancer, personifying it. I ended up talking to it a lot more the rest of the day. "You're never welcome in my body again," I told it. "You're the worst thing to ever happen to me." Swearing at cancer and threatening it made me picture these blobby, bloody masses of tissue cowering in a corner, and I liked that. It needed to cower because I was done and moving on. It needed to be afraid. Cancer had no place here, ever again.

11

THE GOLF LESSON

Connor Jackson

By the start of Tuesday, Katie was sleeping more and feeling worse. She had more visitors with balloons and, now, a big pink flamingo. They were all concerned. During this part of the treatment, we often have to reassure the family that it was the right choice. They'd seen Katie go through chemo already. She's technically cancer-free. Most patients would have already lost all their hair. Katie's thick, curly hair was a real exception.

Unfortunately, Katie's health kept declining all day. We took a blood test once a day, and it took some time to process. Katie's hematocrit was lower than most people's on a normal day, but she was feeling overly weak and becoming paler as the day progressed. When she told me she was seeing stars when she tried to stand up to get to the bathroom, we became even more concerned. The doc ended up calling for a blood transfusion. Now, a blood transfusion is not a comfortable experience. We warm it up so you don't have cold blood entering your veins, but it's still weird, and it's hard on a super-sick person. We don't do these often on our floor.

———

WHILE KATIE WAS FEELING her worst, I was getting into the easy part of the training, although I'd be running a total of thirty miles for the week. My plan called for mostly easy three- or four-mile runs for the next two weeks, with longer runs each Sunday. I'd chosen a few different routes to keep things a bit more fun, including the Buckeye Trail, and in Levi's neighborhood so I could eat dinner at their house after the run.

That day, I changed at work and went right to the Buckeye Trail stream route so I could shower and get to my golf lesson in plenty of time. I wasn't sore anymore and ran my three miles faster than I meant to, so I was home with Pumpkin and the mail by four o'clock.

I struggled with what to wear. "I think golfers wear colorful vests," I told Pumpkin, who had plopped onto my bed. I did not own a vest. Pumpkin watched as I scrutinized my wardrobe, holding up shirts and shorts without putting them on. He knew this was not my normal behavior.

Golfers also wore plain khaki shorts, not cargo shorts, I remembered. I had only one pair of shorts that weren't cargo (or running shorts) that I'd bought for someone's summer wedding. Erin had picked them out for me. They were navy, not khaki, but I figured they'd have to do. I tucked in my green polo shirt. This is not the kind of thing I wear on a casual date or for any sort of lesson, but I felt I needed to play the part. And my running shoes from last summer were not the golfer's spiked shoes I pictured, but that's what I had. Pumpkin seemed to think I looked okay too. He gave me one of his approving, serious cat looks.

———

I DROVE to the golf course parking lot and signed in at the registration desk. A teen with braces and a Park District polo shirt with a name tag that read "Victor" directed me where to sit and wait. I was right about the polos. Everyone was wearing one, Victor included.

I saw Leah before she saw me. She was also in a Park District polo shirt, her long hair held back in a braid. She was wearing a skort and what looked like zoot suit shoes with spikes. They were exactly what I had pictured golfers wearing but looked way cooler on her. When I stood up, she saw me and smiled. She hugged me hello, and I totally went with it. I thought we were starting things off well.

Knowing that I did not own clubs without even asking, Leah brought me into another area to try out and select some golf clubs to rent. She watched as I held some in a stance she directed and decided on a few. We packed them into a bag that I insisted on carrying, although she, as my teacher, was supposed to do that. It was then I realized I had asked her out on a date—at her work. If someone had asked to hang out with me at the nurse's station on my ward, it would have been weird and most certainly *not* a date. And I knew then that I needed to ask her to go out to dinner, too—this did not count.

Leah steered me across the clubhouse and onto what I thought at first was a covered, attached porch. Turned out it was the driving range. She waved hello to a few people, also in Park District polos. I had no idea what I was doing, but Leah was an excellent teacher. She poked fun at me in the nicest of ways, helping adjust my grip, my foot placement, my stance—pretty much everything. I was laughing too and took some practice swings, as instructed.

"Okay, let's do this. You've got a solid swing. I'm putting down the first ball!" she said, trying to pump me up, and then clapped her hands a couple of times. I swung, hit, and watched the ball go much farther than I expected. But it landed two lanes to the left. I heard the guy on my left chuckle under his breath and felt both my blood pressure rise and my face redden.

"Hey, you haven't done this in a lot of years," Leah said, patting me on the shoulder and making eye contact to distract me from our neighbor. The pat felt electric, and I was glad I was already blushing. "That's not a bad first drive at all. We've got a whole bucket of balls, and your first one will probably be the most off course. Let's do some adjusting."

And so we continued. I was glad when the chuckling golfer finished his bucket. I improved as I swung again and again. Leah was very encouraging, but the lesson was not romantic. I was worn out by the end because I was using different muscles than I normally do. Although I was pretty sure this wasn't a date, I felt good. I'd gotten in a second workout and some face time with a pretty lady.

Plus, I didn't feel as awkward around her now that she'd made fun of my poor golfing skills.

We collected our stuff and headed back to the front of the building.

"So, should we make this a regular weekly lesson? What do you think?" Leah asked, looking at me sideways and grinning. I liked the fact that she wanted to see me again.

"I'm sure it would improve my swing," I said. "I have to admit, though, that golf isn't the whole reason I'm here. What time do you get off? Can we get a drink? Ice cream? Maybe dinner?" I was feeling bolder than usual, and the words just fell out of my mouth.

"I like to start with dessert. You were the last thing on my calendar for the day. Let's do ice cream." She was smiling still. "I need to just grab my things in my office. Let's put these away, and I'll meet you back out here in a few minutes."

And so I sat under Victor's glare while I read some gaming blogs on my phone. I considered booking another lesson with him while I was in the lobby, but thought I should see how the ice cream went first.

———

WE ENDED up at the local creamery that also sells lots of fried food. We ordered mozzarella sticks to share and two ice cream sundaes.

"I haven't had mozzarella sticks in a long time," I said. "I've been trying to eat clean during my half-marathon training."

"That takes some major dedication, but I will remind you it was *your* idea to get ice cream, Mr. Half-Marathon!"

"You got me there! I'm not saying they aren't good! Hey, I'm dying to talk about that building with the pole. What did you dig up about it having to do with making electricity?"

"How is that not the first thing you said to me? Yes! So I told you about the maps and the old farms, right?"

I nodded, dunking my second cheesy stick in the marinara sauce.

"Well, the District owns a ton of small parcels and properties around this area. We have an internal database with addresses, maps, pictures, and notes about how each property was purchased or donated or whatever. Details about the parcel and what's on it." She leaned back from the table for emphasis. "The file for that lot has hardly anything in it."

"Hardly anything in it! What?" This was feeling like a genuine mystery.

"There is a picture of the building, but it's pretty old. The trees and brush around it are a lot smaller."

"What did the notes say?" I asked. I had totally abandoned my food at this point.

"Some details about the trail, the largest trees on the lot, and the invasive plant species on the property. We like to document that kind of thing. But only the size of the building, no details. They called it an 'outbuilding.' But nothing about how tall the pole was or when it was built."

THE STORY THAT MADE US STRONGER   73

"But how did you get energy generation from that?" I felt like she was just dancing around my question.

"Oh, right. The map of the property had a square for the building, and the label next to it said 'power booster.' That's all it said."

"'Power booster,'" I repeated, wondering what that meant. "It's not like the pole is a wind turbine or something. How would a tiny building like that make electricity? I've been doing some homework, too," I continued. "I was wondering if the thing on the end of the pole is an instrument to measure wind speed, and I emailed a wind power person about it, but I haven't heard back yet."

"You'll have to tell me what they say. That's an interesting idea." She took another bite of her sundae. "I drove past the building and saw how the door is falling off the hinges now."

"What do you think? I really want to see what's inside." Now I was doing the dancing around. Could I ask her to break in with me? Would I even go through with it? Katie would want me to.

"Yeah, me too..." she trailed off, picking at her thumbnail with the fingernail of her index finger again. We were both quiet, absorbed in our own thoughts for a minute. A felony could get my nurse's license suspended. Breaking and entering just seemed so serious. I really wanted to see what was inside, what the mystery held, but wasn't sure I had the guts to get in.

"So, you remember Katie? My patient, who called you?" I decided to blame it on her. "She thinks I should break into it. You know, because she can't, being stuck in the hospital. But what if you were there, too? If it's on your golf course, wouldn't that be okay?"

"I'm just not sure. It's not exactly *part of* the golf course, just right next to it."

"Last time I was there, I couldn't move the door," I admitted. "I pushed on it, but it didn't want to move when I shoved it."

"Oh, oh, oh! So you have already tried to break in?"

"I wasn't serious about it. I just wanted a peek inside."

And then our sundaes arrived, mine with strawberry ice cream and marshmallow sauce and Leah's with hot fudge and caramel sauces over vanilla ice cream. I wasn't going to let the conversation run out again.

After my first bite, I said, "I think a crowbar would have helped. And this marshmallow sauce is amazing."

She shook her head at me. "I still don't understand your order. Strawberry ice cream with marshmallow sauce? Hot fudge is the best. I don't understand why it doesn't come standard on every sundae!" I almost took offense, but then she distracted me. "So a crowbar. I'm just not sure about breaking in, Connor. I don't know if I'd get in trouble or if they would consider it a nonissue."

"I know, I know. I've been mulling this over for almost a week. Katie said something that really hit me, though. She says that doing something once doesn't define you." I couldn't believe that I was acting as if I had already decided to do it. I wasn't feeling that confident in my head.

She nodded thoughtfully, pulling the spoon out of her mouth slowly as she did. "Okay. I guess that makes sense." She paused. "But committing a crime goes on your permanent record. I'm just not sure if it's a crime if it's kind of your own building. Maybe I should ask my boss? Maybe he'd be okay with me opening it up?"

"Okay. Yeah. When can you ask him?"

"Tomorrow. I'll email him tomorrow," she said with such confidence, while having hot fudge stuck to her top lip.

The rest of our conversation went well. It turned out that Leah also liked cats and had just gotten a gray kitten named Asher a few months ago. We drove separately, so I walked her to her car. I thought about kissing her after our goodbye but was satisfied when she leaned in for a hug. It was a not-date, after all. We made some tentative plans to get a drink on Saturday for a proper date. I had work and cross-training on my calendar but could meet her that night. She promised to text me with any updates from her boss.

When I got home, I realized I had gotten an email earlier that day from a program manager at one of the wind power nonprofits I'd contacted. She thought the picture didn't look like it had anything to do with measuring wind speed, that it might just be a lightning rod.

I didn't like that idea at all. Why would such a small building need a huge lightning rod on an enormous pole? So I poked around the Internet for information on what lightning rods actually do, how big they usually are, and so forth. I discovered that "lightning protection systems" are big business nowadays because of the damage that power surges can do to electronics. Businesses would have to shut down for days if they were struck by lightning.

Maybe the big pole was to protect something really important inside.

I found the League of Lightning Professionals, which seemed to be a trade group for people working with lightning protection systems. I used the Contact Us form and copied my pole picture into it to inquire if they thought it was a lightning rod. Seemed like a good starting point, given that this group was an authority on the subject.

12

THE LATE-NIGHT PLANS

Connor Jackson

On Wednesday, Katie was feeling low, as expected. Unfortunately, she also had an infection from her immune system having been knocked out. It's pretty common but never comfortable. Because of the infection, visitors were limited.

"Let's get you up." She needed help to get out of her hospital bed at this point.

"My man, this is rough. You promise I'm going to feel better next week?"

"Cross my heart," I promised, making notes on my computer about her daily weight. "This is the worst week. Your body is building itself back up."

Settling back into her pink cocoon, Katie said, "I know you have news after your so-called golf lesson." I had to smile at the slow, low air quotes she used for emphasis.

"Vitals are the same as last night. They're not great,

but they'll be better in a few days. I do have news! But I need to know your pain score first."

"Yeah, okay. Is there something bigger you can give me? I'm going with a nine."

"No one should be at a nine, ever. Looks like the Tylenol isn't quite enough. I'll ask the doc to get you some morphine."

"Well, that sounds like it could do the trick," she said, giving me a slow thumbs-up that turned into hair twirling. "Spill the beans on the date, man."

"Okay, okay. So the golf lesson turned into going out for ice cream and mozzarella sticks."

"I could really go for mozzarella sticks," Katie told me, sleepily. "I like that it went beyond golf."

"She had a lot to say about the building," I said, and relayed what Leah knew from the old records and maps. "Leah thinks her boss might let her get inside it to check it out. I'm really hoping I can be there when she does."

"That's cool. I hope so too. We need to know what's inside. I'm still betting on treasure."

Katie's sister is a doctor at the hospital and stopped in that day for a visit. She ended up sitting on Katie's couch all afternoon doing documentation on her laptop. I was glad Katie was allowed a visitor.

Later that day, I got a text from Leah.

Leah: The boss is not cool with opening the building. Says he doesn't see a point in it.

Well, I'm not cool with his answer!

Connor: Me neither!

I let that text sit for a while and got busy with patients. Finally, I responded:

Connor: So what do we do?

Leah: I don't know.

Connor: I know we are supposed to meet for dinner Saturday, but could we just talk on the phone tonight about it?

Leah: Sure—I have spinning. After dinner?

Connor: Yeah. I'm at Levi & Erin's tonight, so 8:00?

Leah: 👍

That night, I drove to Levi and Erin's house after work. I ran my three easy miles around their neighborhood while Juney rode her purple-sparkle bike with me. She's a really fun running partner and chatted away about who lives in the houses we were passing and who had the best swing set and how many kids were in each family. Honestly, she had told me most of this before—but I always needed a refresher. Unfortunately, I had forgotten to bring another Lego Harry Potter bag.

"Alright, alright! I'm ready to run through the sprinkler! Where are the swimsuits?" I said as we walked through the slider from the deck into the kitchen. Clover was jumping up and down with just-turned-five-years-old excitement. We ran around in the backyard for almost an hour, and then I showered and changed back into my scrubs before dinner so as not to get the dining room all wet.

Erin outdid herself with an amazing meal of grilled salmon and asparagus, plus real mashed potatoes. It was difficult to not hit the potatoes hard. Clover isn't a fan of asparagus, so she ate peas instead.

"So, Connor, I hear you're getting drinks with Leah on Saturday," Erin announced to the dining room table, not really to me. She didn't know about the phone call that night.

"Ooooohhh," Clover cooed at the same time Juney asked, "Leah? Spinning Leah?"

"Wow, news travels fast," I told the audience.

"I just heard at spinning this afternoon," Erin told me, meeting my eyes and smiling.

"So, yeah. She gave me a golf lesson yesterday, and we got ice cream after." To that, both girls protested that *they* wanted to go golfing and get ice cream with me, too. "We had a nice time, so we want to see each other again. Like I want to see you guys again. It is a good idea to go putt-putting next time we have a sleepover." This answer satisfied the girls.

"I'm glad you want to see each other again," Levi said. "She seems like good people."

"She *is* good people! I wouldn't invite her to our party if she wasn't!" Erin retorted. Levi nodded in understanding and agreement.

"So what did, uh . . . what did she say about me?" I asked, mixing my mashed potatoes more than necessary.

"That you need more golf lessons!" Everyone had another chuckle at my poor golfing skills. I laughed too. No blushing in this crowd.

———

I LEFT their house after helping clean up the kitchen. I had some time before our phone call and just kept rehearsing what I might say after I got home. I called Leah right at eight.

"Hello, Mr. Half-Marathon!" was how she answered the phone.

"Hello, yourself!" I couldn't come up with a funny response quickly. I never was good at that sort of thing.

"How was your day?" she asked sweetly. I didn't want to make small talk and just pretended she didn't say it.

"I can't get this building out of my head," I answered instead.

"I've noticed," she quipped back. I could hear the smile in her voice.

"Where else can we find out more about it? What can we do?" I asked.

"I think we have all the county files and the information that the previous owners had. No one else seems to know much else. I could make copies of the files, if you want to see them," she offered.

"But what's *in* there?" I asked. "Who knows that?"

"That's the big question, isn't it? I don't know."

"I know breaking in would be illegal, but what else can we do? Who else could give permission to be in there?" I asked, thinking out loud, frustrated.

"My boss's boss? The Park District executive director?"

I jumped at this new idea. The Park District's executive director was a well-known public figure, young but with a grandmotherly demeanor. "Oh! Totally. Alice Fitzgerald could let us in!" I said.

"Well, I don't really know her. It would be kind of

weird to just contact her out of the blue. And if my boss already said no . . ."

"Yeah. You'd be going over his head. That wouldn't be cool," I agreed. Neither of us said anything for a few seconds.

"So breaking in is what we have to do," she said. "There's no other way to get more information that I can think of. There's no one else with information."

"This isn't quite the conclusion I expected you to come to."

"You forget that I've been wondering about this building for months. You're not the only one with it on your mind."

"And Katie! Katie wants to know what's in there, too." This fact that my stem cell replacement patient wanted to know made up my mind. We wouldn't just be doing it for us.

"And Katie," she agreed. "So, do we go during the day? Act like it's part of my job?"

"Well, I don't think you should do anything illegal while you're getting paid by the Park District," I said.

"Yeah, you're right."

"It's a really busy place after work. I think we'd need to go at night."

"That makes sense but makes it sound so much more illegal," she said, and then added in a whisper: "And exciting!"

"Okay. So, when? After drinks on Saturday?" I asked.

"That's too far away!" She must have read my mind.

"I was hoping you'd say that!"

"Tomorrow?" she asked.

"I'm off work, actually. I could go any time! It's dark at nine. How's that?" I asked. What was I getting myself into? Why was I doing this?

"Nine is too early, I think. People might be around still."

"You think?" I asked, not so sure. I was certainly never out on the trail that late.

"I think we need to go late. Like midnight."

"Yeah. That is late. For sure, no one would be around then," I said. And so we made plans to break into the building that I was obsessed with. I was excited but so unsure at the same time.

13

THE DEPRESSION

Katie Brandt

Having cancer was hard. Chemo treatments were hard. But even when I was pregnant and my cancer was at its height, I was not as sick as I was in the stem cell replacement ward. I felt like I wasn't myself for days while my immune system was repairing itself. I couldn't do anything. It was the only time I slept well during my stay, but it was almost as if I were passed out. I didn't dream. I didn't miss my people. I was sort of . . . nothing. Time passed without me knowing it, and I completely lost a few days. I had an infection that made me get up to go to the bathroom a lot, but it was like I was sleepwalking. I'd never have survived without my nursing crew. They deserved all the chocolates we left out, replenished by Rachel and my sisters when they were allowed to visit. I had nothing to do with handing out the chocolate in those days.

When I regained myself, I felt low, sadder and more

helpless than I ever have. I hadn't been outside for weeks and couldn't remember the last time I'd seen someone who wasn't a hospital worker. I was told that Karissa had been there, but I didn't really remember her well. The food was tasteless, even though I was still calling Renee for the real stuff. I felt like such an emotional, worthless lump, such a helpless pile of mush that couldn't take care of myself, let alone my sweet babies. I felt like I was trapped in a damp, sad, dark cave and would never get out. Maybe the cave was the building that Connor and I were so excited about, but its door was covered with hard, packed snow that I couldn't move because it was so thick and cold and I was oh so tired. I was stuck, and the way out felt more than impossible.

Looking back, the point when I said that I couldn't deal with my kids is when my doctor saw that I needed some depression meds.

"This isn't unusual, Katie. You should know that," Connor told me when he gave me my first dose. "The ladies tend to feel lower than guys a lot of the time here."

"What? You're saying depression is sexist?" I asked him.

He chuckled and said, "I just think women get into their own heads more and there's nowhere for the thoughts to go when you're so stuck in a hospital room for weeks." I nodded, taking the pill and water cup. He continued: "There's no shame in helping your body right a chemical imbalance. That's what depression is a lot of the time."

And with just one pill a day, I felt a lot better, felt more myself. The packed snow in front of the dark little building melted slowly, and light trickled in. I can't say the exact day I was lifted out of the building, but I knew I wasn't there anymore. I also knew I wasn't ready to leave the hospital, but I could and I would, eventually. And somehow I knew I wasn't only in the hospital for my kids. Something had shifted in my mind. I was also here to beat cancer for myself. So much of the so-called battle was for PJ, Josie, and Juliet. Yes, I wanted to cuddle my kids again and rest in my husband's arms. So bad. But I also wanted my own life back. I wanted me back. Depression drugs helped me find myself again.

14

THE NOT-A-BREAKING-AND-ENTERING-KIND-OF-GUY BREAKS IN

Connor Jackson

I tried to sleep in on Thursday, but Pumpkin was used to my alarm going off at 6:00 a.m. and kept checking in on me, jumping as heavily on the bed as he could.

Today I'd scheduled a seven-mile tempo run, which meant I'd be running faster during the middle five miles to get my body used to that pace. I left an hour after finishing my morning coffee and cinnamon oatmeal with protein powder, looking forward to the challenge of a good tempo run. I decided that I really needed to run the loop that went by the building. That meant I had to run the route twice, giving me the opportunity to stare it down more often. Its stoic brick walls gave me no response and revealed nothing, as usual.

"I'll see you later," I whispered to it on my second lap.

It was a good run. I probably should have let my breakfast digest longer. While running, I got a few side stitches but massaged them away without a problem. I always run better in the afternoon, but running in the morning left the rest of the day wide open. My iliotibial band along the outside of my right thigh was bothering me a bit, so I did extra stretches and used a foam roller, too.

As I was stretching on my patio, Claire, my neighbor, came over to say hello. We chatted about her garden and the sad potted plants on my patio. At the beginning of the summer, we had gone to our town's local garden center, Patty's Plant Place, where she's a regular. I think of Claire as an adopted grandma. These were my first attempt at growing flowers on my patio, and I did not seem to have a green thumb.

"I think you need to sprinkle some diatomaceous earth in your pots to get the Japanese beetles to leave your flowers alone," she said after closer inspection.

"You know way better than me how to take care of them!" I said. "Do you have any of that stuff?" She laughed and nodded.

I spent the rest of the day doing boring things like laundry and playing video games, and started a new thriller my mom and I had decided to read together. In the afternoon, I heard from the League of Lightning Professionals. They said a lightning rod is not supposed to be installed on a pole like the one on the building. So still no idea about what the pole was for. For dinner, I made a quick curry that I could reheat for lunches over the weekend so I wouldn't have to cook again. Midnight is past my normal lights-out, and I didn't want to be overly tired, but my eyes seemed to be just as excited about the prospect of breaking into the building with Leah as my brain was. Leah and I exchanged a few texts that day.

Connor: I can't believe we're going to break into a building tonight!

Leah: Me neither!

Connor: I'm going to bring a flashlight and a backpack. Seems like a good idea.

Leah: Then we can take pictures and have light at the same time. For sure a good idea.

Connor: I'm just going to walk to the building from my condo. Where do you think you should park?

Leah: Should I park in the lot down the road? Or should I meet you at your place?

I wasn't totally into her coming into my condo at midnight, though I could meet her at the door and just not invite her in. I didn't want to seem like a creep who wanted things to move too fast.

Connor: OK. I'll just meet you outside.

I texted her my address and waited.

———

I WAS SITTING on the couch playing Zelda with Pumpkin Muffin next to me when I heard a car drive into the lot in front of my condo at 11:54 p.m. The headlights beamed into my living room, and the car turned off. Leah had arrived.

I pressed Pause and grabbed my phone and the crowbar I'd left by the door. As I locked the door, I said goodbye to Pumpkin. I rarely address Pumpkin on departure, but it seemed fitting that night.

"So it's midnight," I said as a greeting.

"So it is." She went in for a hug again. "This is crazy! I could get into so much trouble at work!" She was wearing her brown hair in a tall bun on the top of her head, with her bangs swept to the side. We were both wearing hoodies and jeans. She had taken the precaution of putting on hiking boots. As always, I was in old running shoes.

"We can call it off at any time. Right now, we're just going for a midnight stroll. The trail is out back. There's a path from my patio," I said, pointing.

She followed me through my front yard and around the back. My condo is on the end, so I have a bit of a space between my building and the next. There are security lights around the buildings, so we didn't use the flashlight until we were actually on the trail. Once we were there, we kept silent but communicated with nods that she should turn it on and that I should put the crowbar in her backpack. Her flashlight was an older Maglite with big D batteries inside.

We had about a half-mile walk up the trail, which was all uphill. I told her so much in a whisper. It was very different on the trail at night. The woods around it felt deeper, the road farther away. The crickets were louder, as were our soft footsteps on the blacktop. Leah shone the light straight down right in front of our feet. I could see a few bugs in the spotlight and had no notion of the golf course in the distance. We walked in silence, listening.

It was hard to see much in the dark. I spotted the huge

poplar tree on the edge of the trail before I saw the building. And once the building came into view, a movie started in my mind. I could see myself doing something crazy. I could see the archetypal pretty girl and the awkward guy getting into trouble together. What usually happened in a story like that? I couldn't remember. Probably nothing good.

We stopped on the trail next to the building and looked at each other. We had not seen a car on the road near the trail or another person out for a late-night walk. I led the way over to the gate in the fence. The U handle opened a lot easier this time. I had forgotten work gloves, anyway. I pulled the gate toward us and entered, stomping on the vegetation on my way around the building, jeans protecting my legs against the thorns and ivy, unlike my last visit. Leah followed and directed her beam of light ahead of me so I could see where to put my feet.

At the door, we looked at each other again. The gap between the door and its door jamb was unchanged.

"So here we are," she whispered with a smile.

"I'll take a picture. For Katie," I said. It had just occurred to me to document the entire process. I aimed my phone at the door, and what I was doing really began to sink in. Was this right? Was I stalling with the picture? Did I really want to break into a building?

"Let's do this," I said, courage building and allowing me to not whisper anymore. Leah turned around so I could get the crowbar out of her backpack and I did, the zipper louder than it should have been, the crowbar banging against the fence. Every tiny noise sounded like a shout.

I inserted the crowbar on the hinge side of the door and pushed and pulled, pushed and pulled. Splinters and a deep impression of the crowbar showed up in the wood after a few rounds, while the knob and its latch objected. The bottom hinge was off completely when I started, and the screws of the top one began to give way at my pushing and pulling. Leah's light moved up and down the door in slow motion.

After about a minute, I stopped, looked at Leah, and gave a shrug. I shoved my shoulder and all my weight into the middle of the door. The movie in my head slowed as the hinge gave way and the entire door fell away from the doorjamb. Then I was sprawled on the dusty, musty floor in the flashlight's circle, the door to my right side. I heard Leah take a picture.

We were both trying not to yell, but quietly threw around excited exclamations.

"That was too easy!" I yell-whispered, finding my feet and hitting my knees to knock off dust. Leah stepped in as I got my phone out and turned on its flashlight.

15

THE INSIDE

Connor Jackson

The room was tiny, with just enough space for us to fit, along with the built-in table or workbench on the far side and a wooden stool that I hadn't seen before. There were yellowed papers scattered across the table, as well as some still held by a weathered clipboard. The papers were covered in dust that contained charts of numbers written in pencil.

I snapped more photos for Katie.

The ceiling was also made of brick and had wooden beams. In a corner of the ceiling, a circle had been patched over. I shone my light up and down the beams as Leah leafed through the papers. Looking back, I heard a car outside as I was inspecting the ceiling, but thought nothing of it. Unfortunately, the ambient noise of cars doesn't always register in our modern ears.

"This place is really old," I stated. The bricks in the

walls were crumbling, red dust coming off on my sweaty fingers.

Our feet left footprints in the dust, and I felt underwhelmed. I had expected something more from this monument to time. I had expected some answers, an obvious reason why this tiny, abandoned building was standing in the woods with a fence around it and a huge pole strapped to its side.

"No real clues about why it's here, though, what it does . . . or did," Leah said, echoing my thoughts. She knelt down to inspect the underside of the workbench. She ended up lying on her back to get a look at the underside of it, getting dusty.

I also bent down and shone my light on the floorboards. I ran my fingers along the grooves in the wood. There was nothing else to look at, and I was determined to find something: that treasure Katie was expecting. I shone my light on the underside of the stool, hoping for graffiti at least.

"There are wires under here," Leah said. I crawled under the workbench have a look, too.

"Wires. I guess leading to the pole outside?" I mused.

"Yeah, seems like it," Leah agreed. "They're cut, so I guess whatever the pole was for isn't working anymore?" I took another picture.

As I was pushing myself up, my left hand flat on the wood, I felt something different, softer. I turned around again to get a better look.

"What's this?" I asked, trying to find the spot again with my index finger.

"What's what?" Leah asked, and she swung her flashlight over to see—and hit me square in the jaw. I tasted blood in my mouth and saw stars for a second. This lady was strong!

"Oh, no!" Leah yelled and started apologizing profusely.

"There's something here," I tried to say, but my jaw wasn't doing what I wanted. She was too focused on my face and not the soft part of the floor. "I'm really fine," I said thickly. My mouth hurt, but it didn't feel urgent. My teeth seemed intact, at least. Still, she put her hand on my face, and we looked each other straight in the eyes. In another time and place, this could have been romantic. In an actual movie, I'd have gone in for a kiss. Maybe the blood would have been a turnoff? I'm still not sure.

"I'm okay," I said after too long, my cheek already feeling a bit swollen. "Let's see what this is."

Leah took her hand away from my face and aimed her flashlight at a knot of really old rope that seemed inlaid in the wood. It was bristly and kind of hurt my fingertips when I touched it. We looked at each other again.

"Can you pull on it or something?" she asked.

I dug my fingernails into the knot and pried it out. Slowly, a weathered rope followed the knot and after just four inches were above the floor, the rest of the rope caught on something and no more would come out of the hole. I gave it a tug, but nothing happened.

"So there's a hole in the floor with a short rope in it," I said, annoyed. It didn't make any sense to me.

Leah was looking scanning the floor around me.

"Connor! You've got to move out of the way! I think it's the handle for a door—a trapdoor!"

"Wait! What? A trapdoor?" I crawled away from the rope. On my hands and knees, I pulled the rope with both hands, eager to find secrets for Katie.

"Careful!" Leah chided me. She was right. Old rope couldn't be that strong. I nodded, and pulled more gently, more slowly.

After the puff of dust settled, we could now see the outline of a square on the wooden floor. I pulled more, but without force; I didn't think the inlaid wood would come up.

"Let's try to get some of the dirt out of the cracks," I said, wiping the edges of the trapdoor with my fingers. "It seems stuck." Talking didn't really feel great with my cheek still throbbing.

Leah produced a pen from her bag and dug at the spaces between the boards. I found the crowbar and did the same. After our work, the outline of the trapdoor was much more apparent. Leah put her palms flat on the wood and tried to shift it back and forth, and we saw movement.

"Looks loose! Okay. I'll try again." I pulled softly on the old rope, then harder, but nothing happened.

"Not loose enough," she said and then stood up and stomped on it, making more dust fly in my face. "Sorry," she whispered.

"It's okay," I said, coughing a bit, but really not caring because I could feel the door shift this time as I was pulling. Coughing also made my swollen face hurt. I adjusted my hands so that they were closer to the wood, at the opposite end of the rope from the knot. This time it was moving.

Leah got the crowbar and nudged at the side of the trap door, too. We slowly worked it free. With a thump, the panel of wood came away from the floor. The short rope had another ancient knot on the other side of the wood that I could see now was holding it in place. It was good that I was careful with it.

I was beside myself with excitement. We'd just opened a trapdoor! A trapdoor! I looked at Leah, and she was smiling with all her teeth showing.

She directed her flashlight into the hole, and I used my phone's flashlight. It was the basement I had imagined before, with a dirt floor, but it wasn't as deep as I'd expected. All over that dirt floor were glass jugs arranged in neat rows.

"Not exactly the treasure Katie was thinking of, huh?" I asked. To say I was disappointed wasn't quite right. My extreme excitement had passed and had been replaced with curiosity. What was this place? Why were there so many jugs? Was this a stash during Prohibition?

Without a word, Leah swung her legs into the hole and edged herself down into the basement. Her head and shoulders were still above the trapdoor once her feet hit the floor. She crouched down, her flashlight helping her see more below, and said, "So, so dirty under here."

Leah moved below the floorboards and took her light with her, so I was mostly in the dark. I hopped down too, crouching to get a better look at the bottles and the room. Leah was a few feet away from me, exploring. I felt claustrophobic and didn't want to be in such a low space.

Instead, I picked up the bottle nearest me and inspected it. It was a thick glass: heavy and wavy. I could tell it was old. I put it back down and took a step into the creepy room because a jug three away had something in it, and I wanted to see what it was.

16

THE PAPER

Connor Jackson

I edged closer to the bottle. I had to stoop low and creep along slowly. Leah was in my peripheral vision, practically skipping around this dank, low-ceilinged basement. She was shorter than me but still couldn't walk upright. When I got to the bottle I wanted, I picked it up and made my way back to the hole in the ceiling as fast as I could.

"I think there are thirty-six jugs, two cracked, thirty with stoppers. And a wooden crate filled with these pointy metal things, with some tools. Also, fifty-four metal pails all stacked together," Leah reported. She was holding up one of the pieces of metal, about the size of my palm, and had kicked the pails for emphasis. "Plus a few tattered blankets. And lots of mouse poop."

"Yeah. Lots of mouse poop," I said as I turned the bottle upside down and shook it. This was one of the bottles with a stopper. "I found something interesting. It looks like a piece of paper." But it was stuck to the bottom inside the jug. After a bit more jostling, it came free. Leah had joined me standing up in the trapdoor. We were standing really close to each other, and I couldn't help but feel a bit more excited.

"A message in a bottle?" she joked, watching my progress.

It wasn't as easy as I thought to get the stopper off. Then I couldn't get my fingers inside the jug to get the paper out.

"I can try," Leah offered. I handed over the jug. Her smaller fingers could reach inside better, and she held it between her index and middle fingers. For some reason, she handed it directly to me.

The next few minutes lasted an hour. Looking back, I can see the whole thing play out as if from a drone overhead.

Outside there were suddenly sirens and red-and-blue flashing lights. Our eyes met, and Leah froze, with her hand still inches above mine. I held the paper in my hand and hadn't gotten a good look at it yet.

"Um. So. Uh," Leah stammered.

"I guess . . . the police?" I replied, fear hitting me like a wall. But Leah became resolute and stood up straighter.

"Okay. You close up here, and I'll see what's going on outside." She picked up her flashlight and backpack and crawled out of the trapdoor. Moving toward the door, she faced the consequences boldly.

I shoved the paper in my pocket and pulled myself

out of the basement. My mind was racing, and it killed me not to unfold the paper, not to see what it was, but I knew I couldn't yet. Acting on instinct, I threw the crowbar into the basement before replacing the wooden door cover. I used my foot to mess up the dust more to hide the wooden panel. I made sure the top rope knot was tucked into its hole in the wood. I was worried. I didn't want to be in a ton of trouble. In a panic, I somehow sent a text to Levi before I got to the door.

Connor: I think I'm in trouble, bro.

Leah was already outside the fence, talking with a policewoman. Another police car pulled up behind the first one as I stepped out of the building. I could hear Leah explaining that she worked for the Park District and we were just out for a walk and wanted to see what was in the building. Making my way out of the fence was a lot easier with the trampled vegetation this time.

"I'll need both of your driver's licenses," the police-woman said when I came up next to Leah. She was very matter-of-fact and stone-faced. I really don't even know why I had my wallet in my pocket to begin with.

We handed them over, and the other officer joined us, a guy with a ginger mustache like a cop would have in a movie. I could feel my phone vibrate in my pocket with what I expected was Levi's response. I still don't know why he was awake at that time of night. I wished I could give him more details but didn't dare. I was kicking myself for not figuring out what the consequences of breaking and entering were in Ohio. A felony might mean I'd lose my nursing license. I started sweating thinking about that.

The policewoman stared me down and started questioning me. "So Mr. Jackson, what's your story? Ms. Alger here tells me she works for the Park District and just wanted a peek inside this building. It's an odd time of night to be out just taking a stroll."

"That's the story, officer. I live off of the trail down there," I agreed, pointing toward my condo complex, knowing she couldn't see it. I was thankful my mouth was working better, but I still didn't sound right. I'm not sure if either of the police officers noticed. "We were on a walk and wanted to see inside. The door was already broken." I knew I was talking too much and shut my mouth hard, which hurt. Leah nodded in agreement.

"I'll be back," the policewoman announced. She went to her car and started typing on her laptop. I could see her making references to our driver's licenses.

The mustachioed policeman had yet to say anything; he just stood a few feet away from us in a wide stance, his thumbs in his pockets.

"I'm really sorry I got you into this," I whispered to Leah.

"Not your fault. I wanted to see too."

The policeman shook his head at us to indicate we should stop talking. So we stood and waited for what felt like a half hour. I could feel more texts go off in my pocket. I wanted to ask our guard if I could look at my phone, but I figured he'd be unhappy with it.

Finally, the policewoman came back and nodded to her colleague. "I'm going to have a look inside the structure," she said. And so the three of us watched her wend her way through the fence and into the building. With her flashlight moving around inside, the door really lit up, and I could see why the car that passed on the road would have called the police. I realized I was holding my breath and didn't want her to find the trapdoor, the jugs, and my crowbar. I didn't want the authorities to really know the contents of the building. I wanted the discovery to be ours for a while, a secret.

She wasn't in the building long, maybe two minutes. We all watched her progress back. Once she was in our huddle again, she stated with no feeling, "I'm sure you both know that trespassing is a criminal offense." We nodded. The red-haired policeman nodded, too. I looked at the ground. Leah started picking at her thumbnail with her forefinger again. "I probably could take you downtown and book you, but I won't. Not much in there. No personal property harmed. You didn't steal anything. This building is abandoned, after all." She handed us our licenses and took her notebook out of her pocket. "I'm writing up criminal citations for both of you. You will have this citation on your permanent records, and misdemeanors if you either plead guilty or are found guilty. You will call this number at the bottom for a date to appear for an arraignment. Is that clear?"

I felt numb but still managed to nod. "Not the breaking and entering kind of guy" had earned himself a misdemeanor and a trip to court for trespassing. I tried to study the piece of paper she'd handed me, but none of the words made sense yet. At least she had circled the phone number at the bottom of the page.

"We'll make sure this gate is secure by morning. I will

drive you back to Mr. Jackson's house. Down the trail," she said, her manner teasing but her face still serious.

The policeman drove away, and we got into the back of the first police car. We were all silent. Leah's hand found mine, and she held my hand for the short ride. I was glad to not be alone too.

17

THE MAP

Connor Jackson

After the police car drove away, I was obligated to ask Leah inside to see what was in my pocket. I was a middle schooler yet again, and awkward about it. Yes, I wanted this relationship to move further, but this was not the night to do it, and how did I make it clear while still inviting her to my place in the middle of the night?

"I didn't clean up or anything," I apologized as I unlocked the front door. Both my video game and Pumpkin were right where I left them at midnight. It was after one in the morning now. Leah did that thing that everyone does when they're in a house for the first time, looking the walls up and down, inspecting the furniture and décor—taking it all in. The dirty dishes in the sink and groceries half put away glared at me.

I rushed her over to the dining room table and dug out

the treasure gently. "I think it's a piece of paper," I said, turning on the light over the table. Instead of placing it on the surface, I put it into her ready, cupped hands.

"Hold on! A picture!" I said and found my phone. It was full of texts from Levi and Erin. They would have to wait. I took a pic of the paper in her hands.

Ever so gingerly, she unfolded it. Dust and grey flecks fell onto the table. It cracked a bit on the third crease, yellowed paper specks joining the dust on the table.

Once unfolded, the paper was by no means flat. She held it by opposite corners and laid it on the table, carefully, slowly. There was no way we would flatten it out without cracking it further.

"So it's a map," I said, looking from the crumbling paper to Leah.

"A really old one."

I took another pic to show Katie. We studied it together in silence.

The ink was faded, navy where I assumed it used to be black. The whole paper was square, a bit over a foot on each side. The map depicted a wooded place with big rocks, conifers, and deciduous trees drawn in. There was a simple compass rose pointing north with a path winding north to south. The map seemed to focus on the path, with milestones such as a farmhouse with pigs and cows, a stream, an oak tree, an interestingly shaped rock, and near the top, a little building on a hill with a poplar tree next to it. Each tree had its leaves drawn next to it in detail. There were filled-in triangles next to both the building and the farmhouse.

"This is our building!" I yell-whispered, pointing to the poplar tree and brick structure.

"No way!" Leah yell-whispered back. We smiled at each other.

"This is crazy! What do we do with it?" I asked, no longer whispering, realizing that I didn't need to whisper in my own home.

Leah was talking over me. "What a find! I bet this is like two hundred years old!"

"It feels worth a misdemeanor right now!"

"It does!"

We settled down and stared at it longer.

"I wonder why there was a map to a path in the middle of the woods? There are no towns on it, no roads," Leah finally said.

"Yeah, for real," I agreed, yawning.

"And seriously, how do we keep it from crumbling more?"

I was nervous that Pumpkin would get on the table and mess with it, so we settled on transferring the map carefully to my largest cookie sheet, putting it in the office, and closing the door. This meant that Leah passed the pink guest room and had to get the explanation about Juney and Clover. I put Pumpkin's scratching post in the hallway.

I had to get up in a few hours and said a quick goodbye to Leah. I don't kiss and tell, but yeah, there was a kiss involved.

———

HERE ARE the texts I had to deal with after she left:

LEVI: Dude, what's up? How are you in trouble?

...

Not responding is not a good sign.

...

You're really making us really worry.

Then Erin got into it in our group chat and started with the sisterly threats.

Erin: What are you doing up after 12 p.m.? This is so not cool to send such a cryptic text to Levi! What's up? We're going to kill you if you don't respond!

Connor: I'll tell you more later. I am going to bed, but I was worried I might end up in jail tonight. Leah & I broke into a building and found an old map.

———

I GOT UP AS LATE as I could without being late to work. There were plenty more texts from all interested parties, including Leah, and I tried to respond between getting dressed and eating breakfast. I was lucky I'd already packed the curry and could just throw into my lunch bag.

After I parked with a few minutes to spare, I texted Ed to make sure we were still on for our four-miler after work on the Buckeye Trail. We were set to meet at a trail-head that was about halfway between our houses. He was good to go. I told Levi and Erin that I'd be at their house for pizza after the run, knowing that they were going to give me the third degree.

Katie was still acutely ill, but the worst part of her recovery was coming to an end. She was sleeping most of the day, except when we woke her up every two hours for vitals. Her body was healing: her color and vitals were both improving. And she was as enthusiastic about the pictures as I'd known she would be. Then I told her about the police showing up.

"Look at you, having a run-in with the law! Oh, man, I wish I could have been there! I'm not shy around the Po Po," she said, with just a little more excitement than the last time I saw her.

"I'm sure you would have been a lot more forward than I was with the police. I was just so freaked out and excited about finding the paper."

"Let me see the picture again. I'm going to take a picture of it." Hospital policy didn't allow us to share phone numbers.

"Good idea! Do you have any ideas about it?" I asked her.

"I'm too tired to come up with anything, but don't worry. It's totally on my mind. I will." I knew she would.

The rest of the day was pretty uneventful beyond the solid nap I took on my lunch break in the on-call lounge.

I called Leah on my way to meet Ed, and we firmed up plans for drinks—and now a full dinner—on Saturday. I told her about Katie's excitement, and we agreed we had both been distracted all day by thoughts of a two-hundred-year-old map hiding from my cat in my office.

I was sluggish on the run and glad we weren't going

farther than four miles. Ed's slower pace felt good. I started to tell him about the building, but when he thought I was insane for even thinking about breaking in, I didn't tell him the rest. He might have been right. Insanity might have been the problem.

18

FURTHER DISCOVERIES

Connor Jackson

I often join Levi's fam on Friday for pizza and movie night, but tonight was different from our norm, because the grown-ups were eating in the kitchen while the girls watched a show in the basement with their pizza and Howie the dog, who was probably also eating some pizza without Levi's permission.

Levi and Erin were really pissed about the text I sent at midnight without a full response or explanation. After I told them the whole story, though, they were on board. I'd known they would be. Erin was ready to drive over to my house to see the map in person that night. She was not satisfied with seeing it on the small screen. Levi was trying to figure out how to pair my phone with the family room TV when Erin realized something I hadn't. She was looking at her own phone because I'd texted her a copy to study while Levi fiddled with the TV.

"I think this map is for someone who is illiterate," she

said, as though making a final decision. "There are a lot of details here without a single written word. The only letter is the N for north."

"N for north. Wow! You're right!" I said, looking over her shoulder. Levi came back over, having given up on the TV.

"So someone with ink and paper who probably *could* read and write made a map for someone who *couldn't*," Levi added, completing Erin's thought. She looked up at him and smiled.

"You guys are geniuses!" I said, standing up. "Except I just realized that we could put the map on the TV with Erin's phone instead of mine." We looked at it on the big screen for a few minutes before the girls came back upstairs.

Then we watched the new Spiderman movie together. Levi made popcorn at intermission. I texted Leah about our new suspicion while snuggling with Clover, who fell asleep before the big fight scene. I was dozing, too.

19

THE TRIANGLES

Katie Brandt

Travis and the kids were long in bed, and I still couldn't sleep. Nothing new. I found myself awake and staring at the lights on my wall, beyond the pictures, beyond the blue heart my nephew Luke had made me, beyond the wall. Just staring. I got up and did a lap around the hospital floor. No one else was stirring. The night-shift nurse, Zofia, gave me a knowing nod as I passed her station.

As I walked, I thought about how my little girls came into this world.

By the time we were twenty-seven weeks into the pregnancy, we had a cesarean session scheduled for thirty-five weeks. Most pregnancies go forty weeks, and twins are considered full term at thirty-seven weeks, rarely making it to thirty-eight weeks. I liked having such a definitive plan. Thankfully, my last round of chemo was canceled because I was feeling so good. We could tell that it was working, so we could wait to do another round of chemo after the girls arrived, when it would be more effective. It felt like a rest and a relief to skip that last chemo. I felt huge and tired, and commuting to the city with my mom for the treatment was always a daylong ordeal. I just wanted to be at home with PJ and relish the remainder of his only-childhood.

The doctors expected the girls to go right into the neonatal intensive care unit once they were born, since they were going to be so small. I was not allowed to breast-feed because of the cancer and all the drugs that remained in my system.

April 11, the date of our scheduled cesarean, finally arrived. Scheduling a time to get babies cut out of your body is very different from how most women experience childbirth. Instead of aiming for a due date, you know the exact time and day. That worked for me because I liked to plan things.

PJ stayed with Travis's cousin, Alyssa, who would bring him to the hospital in the afternoon. We got there early, at 6:30 a.m. Travis was jittery, but I was feeling excited. My mom and dad and my doctor-sister, Karissa, all met us in the waiting room.

"Brandt," the nurse called out to the room, as if there might be someone else there. We were the only family waiting.

Karissa, Travis, and I stood up and met her at the door. The nurse took us to another sort of waiting room where I disrobed and got into one of those thin, cold hospital gowns that never cover enough of my body. They took some vitals and attached an IV to my port. I sat on the edge of a table to get my spinal block.

Travis held my hand as they wheeled me down the cold hallway to the surgery room. Karissa was wearing her scrubs, looking as if she were prepping for the surgery herself. She, my OB (Dr. Heather Malar), and a third high-risk OB were all there, crowding the room with more people than I expected. Someone was at my head, rubbing it and encouraging me. There were a few nurses, a surgical tech, and my oncologist, too, making four doctors present.

They draped my lower body so Travis and I couldn't see what was going on down there. I felt hot, and I was nervous too. I felt a lot of tugging and before I was really ready, "Baby A," Juliet Kora, was crying, and her bloody little body was resting on my chest. She was tiny, just over four pounds, but perfect. So perfect! Each girl had one of my sisters' names as a middle name.

"Baby B," Josie Karissa, was higher up in my body, and Dr. Malar said she had to really stick her arm up in there to pull her out. This girl was just under four pounds, but identically immaculate.

Karissa took pictures for us. My favorite is the one of Travis holding them both in his arms with an enormous grin on his face—super-proud daddy.

Both babies' measurements, temperatures, blood work —everything!—came back without a single issue. They did not have to go into the NICU.

My other sister, Kora, and her son, Luke, were waiting for us when they carted us into our hospital room. Apparently, Luke was so excited to meet these new cousins that he was waiting for her with his coat and shoes on when she walked out of the bathroom after her shower.

PJ visited us that afternoon with Alyssa, who had helped me a lot during my pregnancy. He sat on my lap, cradling both girls with Travis's help, and said in his tiny two-year-old voice, "My babies are here! My sisters!" and I just sobbed. My babies were finally here, and they were healthy. We were all somehow okay; I didn't expect that day to go so easily. I didn't know what to expect, but a clean bill of health for tiny babies of a mom with cancer was not it.

I painted their toenails different colors—purple and teal—to tell them apart on the day they were born. They wore purple and teal hats for the first couple of weeks of their lives. Years later, I still assign them those colors. Juliet is teal, and Josie is purple.

We all recovered for a couple of days in the hospital and were thrilled to get home to be a family of five. My parents, in-laws, sisters, cousins, aunts and uncles, and friends and neighbors all stormed over to our house with food and presents. The girls were so rarely put down with all these people clamoring to hold them, and so strongly loved from the second they arrived at home. PJ had such a great time with all the company, too. I was glad for the help because I felt tired, but not as bad as I had felt while pregnant. My cousin's wife and her daughter even came and spent the night a few times so I could sleep through the night and not wake on the newborn feeding schedule.

Back in my room at the stem cell replacement ward, without my babies, I stood at the window with the overhead light off. The hospital sat on a hill, and I had a wonderful view. I could see all the streetlights and a few cars going slowly by below my window. There was a university across the street, with pretty landscaping and lots of illuminated walking paths and lit windows. A few clusters of students ambled along the paths. Beyond the campus, I could see tall buildings that were probably offices. And farther away, I glimpsed the lights of smaller towns and lots and lots of trees. I wondered if the abandoned building was nestled among those trees on the Park District trail. I was looking in the right direction, anyway, and imagined it was. I picked out a point in the forest and decided that was its location.

I turned on the light over my bed and got out my laptop. Without even gliding over Facebook or my email, I went straight for the map that included the building.

"What else can you tell me?" I asked it. "What are you hiding from me?" I had saved a copy of the photo of the map on my computer and put it next to the modern map with the new buildings and streets and the golf course. I tried to figure out where the trail on the old paper map would fit among the streets currently in the same area. There really wasn't much beyond the golf course and the edge of a housing development.

"What do these triangles mean?" I asked the room. And so I searched for map legends. I searched for historical map legends. I found academic journals studying and documenting old maps, and even a few maps that resembled the one Connor and Leah found in the building. And hours later, I had some ideas to share the next day with my fellow researcher.

20

THE DATE

Connor Jackson

I had to work on Saturday, and Katie turned a big corner. Her white blood cells had factually increased. Her infection was nearly gone. We gave her the okay to have visitors again, and they *all* showed up. I don't think our attending doc expected the deluge of people and maybe would have given it another day, had he known. I saw her parents again, her husband, that pretty doctor-sister whose picture was plastered on one of the elevator doors to our floor, her other sister, and the cousin with red hair. Kids were not allowed to come into our ward, or I'm sure I would have met her children. Katie introduced me to those I hadn't already met, but I can't tell you who they were. We had to remind the droves that she was only allowed to have three people at a time in her room, so some hung out in the waiting room. More dry-erase-marker messages crowded onto her window, making it almost hard to see the street below.

The night before, Katie had done some research and had a huge lead on the triangles next to the structures on the map. We had a tiny conversation while visitors shuffled from her room to the waiting room. She suspected the triangles might be an old-fashioned signal of safe shelter, like a modern-day hotel review. Triangles marked next to fences, trees, or other permanent milestones on a map would tell future travelers that they were safe places to spend the night.

So our little building was a safe place. I liked this idea a lot. I texted Levi and Erin the idea, but wanted to wait until our date tonight to tell Leah.

———

AFTER WORK, I went to the YMCA for a cross-training day and swam thirty laps. During the middle twenty-six laps, I pushed myself on the way down and went slower on the way back. Sort of a tempo swimming workout. I had to concentrate to keep track of the laps, so it wasn't as boring as the elliptical. With all the counting, I wasn't able to ponder our building research at all. But I needed to order yet another accessory to keep my hair out of my eyes, this time a swimming cap.

Leah and I were set to meet at six thirty at a pretty fancy local Mediterranean restaurant. No polo this time, but a button-up shirt with dark jeans and dress shoes. As I got dressed, I realized this first date was unique: Leah and I had already been through some pretty exciting stuff together.

By the time I arrived at 6:32 p.m., Leah had already

gotten us a table and was giving off some irritated vibes. She was leaning back in her seat and had her arms crossed. She said nothing, and I didn't want to stir up trouble, so I just leaned down and hugged her awkwardly. Her return hug had less strength than she'd offered before. She did not stand.

"I was worried you weren't going to show up," she said as I pulled away and sat.

"Oh, well, I certainly wouldn't miss dinner with you," I blurted out. I didn't really want to say that two minutes didn't seem like enough to get mad about. She sat forward, finally, and I pulled her hand across the table to hold it.

"I like to be early, and when people are late, I get nervous," she said with just a bit less chill.

"I guess I'm not always precisely on time and don't worry about a few minutes," I said.

"I'd just appreciate a text or call or something if you're running late."

"Sure," I said, hoping that would end the subject.

We ordered drinks, and they brought us pita and oil for dipping with hummus. After some pleasantries, I told her Katie's theory about the triangles. She was excited about the progress but then dropped some big news.

"So my boss—Warren—called me today. On my day off. He had heard about 'someone' breaking into the building on the edge of the golf course two nights ago." Leah didn't use air quotes like Katie, but her inflection inferred them.

"He heard? Like, the police told him? Did he know it was you and me?"

"He heard from our executive director, Alice Fitzgerald. He didn't say anything about anyone from the Park District being involved. I don't know why the police would have left that detail out."

"Yeah, it's not like either of them were friendly and wanted to help us out."

"I think Warren just didn't want me to hear from someone else about the break-in. But here's the thing," she said, pausing her pita mid-dip in the hummus. "Seems like the building really had her attention. Alice thinks the building should be torn down."

"Wait! What? Torn down?"

"My boss says she thought it already had been. It doesn't have a purpose now and is a 'public hazard' or 'attractive nuisance' after some, you know, *random people* broke into it."

"What? A public hazard? And what's this about it not having a purpose now? As if they knew the purpose before? More than what the database said?" I was feeling like a detective again.

"We're on the same wavelength, Mr. Half-Marathon. I caught that too and really tried to get more info on that bit. But he wanted to get off the phone. I'll see what else I can find out Monday. We have a managers' meeting later this week at the HQ, too, so I'll see the ED in person."

"Okay. And it's not like they'd tear it down tomorrow, right?"

"No way. We move way slower than that. It'd be a month from now, maybe, at the soonest. Or when the golf course is closed for the season."

"So we have some time. I mean, *I* don't think it should be torn down," I said, wondering what purpose it could really have anymore. My adventure with the structure lent it a personal meaning for me, but maybe the the actual owners wouldn't agree, even if they knew about the hidden room and the map. Who am I to say that it didn't need to be torn down?

"It has historical significance!" Leah said, instantly dispersing my doubt with her enthusiasm.

Our waiter came to take our order: stuffed grape leaves for her and falafel for me, with an extra side of baba ghanoush because I can eat baba all day long.

Once he left, Leah continued her thought. "That map, the triangles on it prove that the building was a waypoint. I mean, I don't think just any old building gets triangles like that. I've been thinking about this since we first found it. I think it could be part of the Underground Railroad."

"That totally goes with Erin and Levi's ideas about the person who drew the map and who would be using it. Yeah. Underground Railroad."

"I don't know how we'd ever confirm it."

"Well, I wonder how Katie found the info about the triangles? Maybe that symbol was mostly used by runaway slaves? And what did they call the people who helped them?" I asked, trying to remember middle school history.

"Conductors."

"Right. Maybe the triangles were a code used by runaways and conductors. She didn't really tell me where she found out about their meaning."

"But what this theory doesn't answer is why the big pole and the wires are there," Leah said thoughtfully.

"Yeah, it's not like they had electrical wires back then." We both sat a minute, thinking and chewing on pita. "You know, before I was all gung ho about breaking into the building," I continued, "I was thinking I should just ask my next-door neighbor, who's lived in our condo complex since it was built. It's only about twenty years old, but maybe she would have some idea?"

"But how long has the trail been there? It's in the middle of the woods. Would she have noticed the pole and the building if there hadn't been a trail?"

"You can see the pole from the condos. It's on the top of a hill. So even if the trail wasn't there, I think she would have been aware of it," I said, thinking about Claire and how she often walked her little dog on the trail.

"I can try to find out when that particular trail was built."

"Yeah. And I'll ask Katie about the triangles. We both have homework to do." We smiled at each other, and the conversation turned. Somehow Leah roped me into trying a spinning class with her the following Saturday. It worked with my cross-training schedule, but I was prepared to again look like an oaf. We stayed at the restaurant way past dessert and walked around the neighborhood for a while before parting for the night.

21

THE ANTENNA

Connor Jackson

The next day, I knocked on Claire's door in the early afternoon when I knew she'd be home from church, before I began my thirteen-mile run. Her little Yorkie, Mavis, announced that she was not happy to receive visitors. Claire had a smile on her face when she answered the door, though. I was invited in and offered cookies, as usual. It's impossible to pass up Claire's cookies.

It turns out that Claire had worked out what had happened. She had always noticed a lot while not being nosy. She had seen a car come to my house at midnight because she's always up late reading. Then she read a police bulletin in the newspaper about the building on our trail being broken into the same night. She said she knew it was me but didn't want to bother me to ask.

"You got me. It was me and a friend. Did the paper say I was given a . . . criminal citation? I need to show up to court in two weeks to find out what kind of fine or community service I need to perform."

"The report did mention that. What did you find inside the building?"

I liked her directness. "Not much, really, It's been abandoned for a long time. There was a workbench and some papers. And a stool." I didn't want to get into the map and jugs with Claire. I probably should have. She would have loved it!

"I always wondered what they left in there."

"I was wondering if you knew when it was abandoned and what the building used to do. And who were 'they'?"

"Well, 'they' are the Park District, of course. They used to park a truck there once a week or so to check in on the building and the antenna. I'd see them on my walks on the trail."

"Antenna! Oh, man! I've been wondering what was at the end of the pole! Totally!" She smiled at me, perhaps surprised by my enthusiasm. Then I asked, "But, uh, why did they need an antenna? And what were they checking on? When did it stop working?"

"Something about wave radio. I don't really know, honestly." I stood up straighter, excited. I didn't want to interrupt her, but I had finally gotten to the bottom of it. Shortwave radio! She continued, "And, golly, I'm not sure when they stopped using it, Connor. It was working when I moved in, shortly after Owen died." I nodded in under-standing. She'd told me many times how she sought out a condo after her husband died unexpectedly before the age of sixty. "It got hit by lightning at least ten years ago."

"Really? The pole got hit by lightning?"

"Yes, that's when it stopped working. It was a really bright flash of light and so loud. It surprised me that there wasn't a fire. They tried to fix it, I guess, and then never came back. You should talk to Richard, who goes to my church. He's a HAM radio operator and would know all about this sort of wave radio stuff. He has a huge antenna on his own house."

"Oh, yeah? Richard?"

"He lives in the next development over. They bought their house because it's so high on the hill."

"The building is really up on a hill, too. It makes so much sense that it was an antenna," I said thoughtfully.

"Sure was," Claire agreed, smiling. She offered me another cookie, and I begged off. After she gave me Richard's number, we exchanged stories about her grand-kids and my nieces. She told me the latest gossip about our neighbors across the parking lot who have sunflowers in pots that have grown up to the second-story windows. I also helped change the batteries in her thermostat.

After about an hour, I went back home and prepared for thirteen miles. I downed a banana with peanut butter and drank a big glass of water. I changed into my running clothes and packed an energy gel in my shorts pocket. I had planned to do that for the race, and since this was a bit of a preview, I wanted to make sure I'd be happy with the results. I hadn't run this far in a long time. Eleven miles had left me sore the previous week, and I didn't want to feel as bad this time. I also decided to just try a baseball cap again for hair management. After one last bathroom break, I headed over to the Buckeye Trail. I drove to the two-thirds of the run mark and stashed a water bottle under a bush. Then I did some jumping jacks to warm up my muscles and went through my stretching routine, doing extra IT band stretches and double counts for the rest—and I was off.

The miles went faster than I expected. I felt stronger than I had the week before. I sucked the gel down at mile seven, which helped break up the time. It might have helped. I left the wrapper in my pocket. I was glad for the hidden water, too. The hat worked well enough. I ended up turning it backward, which wasn't the plan, but my hair was out of my eyes. The bottom of my feet were aching by the end, but not my legs. And I saw a heron hanging out in the water as I crossed the bridge over the stream. What's crazy was that the heron and I totally made eye contact.

When I got home, I iced my feet again, drank electrolytes, and took ibuprofen as a precaution. Pumpkin played with the ice while I texted Leah, Levi, and Erin about Claire's intel. I wished I had Katie's number. An antenna and another lead! Exciting stuff. But a nap seemed essential, so I decided to call Richard another day.

————

SURPRISINGLY, I really wasn't feeling that sore the next day. My feet still felt a bit hot, so I wore my running shoes to work.

And Katie was feeling even better than the last time I'd seen her, two days before. Her lab result numbers were all increasing and looking great. I could tell that she'd had a lot of visitors on my day off. She had three containers of homemade cookies, and the candy bowl that Katie provided as an awesome patient was overflowing with new varieties. I allowed myself to take a few more than I usually would.

After Katie's morning weigh-in and vitals, she asked eagerly, "How's the training? Any building updates?"

"Yeah. Going well. Feeling good."

"How many miles was your long run this week?"

"Thirteen! The race is less than two weeks away!"

"You're going to be so ready, my man!"

"Thanks. I'm feeling great." I told her the news from Claire.

She was delighted. "This is big! We finally know what they used it for! But we still don't know its long-term history—the jugs, the map, that is."

"I think I'll call Richard on my lunch break. Seems like I should visit him in person. I'll try to set up a meeting when I call," I said, as she settled into the bed again.

"I can call him if you want."

"Always ready to make a phone call!" I said. "No, we know him through my neighbor. I should be the caller."

"Alright. I'm really into the idea of the building being both an antenna *and* a safe place for runaway slaves. Such a helpful little square of bricks."

"'Helpful little square of bricks!' I love it!"

I called Richard on my lunch break. Claire had told him I'd be calling, apparently. Maybe she was being nosy this time. I told him about our little building and its antenna and that I wanted to know more about its uses when it was active. He ended up inviting me over to see his HAM radio setup. I'd visit the next day. After some discussion in our group text, Erin encouraged me to bring him a six-pack of local beer. That seemed like a good idea.

After work, I went straight to the rec center with my gym bag without an actual plan. I ended up in the big cardio room and did a bit of circuit training. After warming up for five minutes on the treadmill, I tried the stair-stepper for another five and then pushed it on the bicep curl machine. I went around the room trying different machines, but didn't leave it all on the gym floor.

When I got home, Erin was asking via text to video-chat. After I got on, Juney wanted to talk about school starting on Wednesday. I felt for her. The end of summer vacation was hard! We ended up planning our sleepover for Saturday night, and I promised to come over after school on Wednesday, too. The start of the school year also meant that Clover was going back to day care instead of having a sitter when Erin was working. Chloe told me she loved her "school" and was excited to see her friends. No drama there!

22

THE SUGAR SHACK

Katie Brandt

I spent a lot of time staring at the photos on my walls in the hospital. Every night when Travis got home from work, he and the kids would play in the living room and I'd video-chat with them for hours. Josie and Juliet were tiny and had no idea what was going on, but it was good to see them every day. PJ didn't really seem to understand that I was on the TV. He was only two, but he'd talk to me as if I were there. We also had a screen in his room, so I could read a story and say a prayer with him before bed. I'd often wake up at night and just stare at his sleeping shape under the covers. I did a lot of staring.

One night, as I was watching his little chest rise and fall, it hit me why the little building we were so excited about looked familiar. It wasn't the shape of it or even the building material; it was its placement.

My Grandpa Marsh had owned a lot of land, much of it forested. My sisters and I spent many hours exploring those wooded acres with him while he identified wild-flowers, birds, animal tracks, and trees for us. He also had a grove of sugar maple trees with a sugar shack next to them. Every few years, we were at his house at the right time for making syrup. We'd help tap the maple trees with metal spiles to harvest the sap, which slowly leaked into steel pails. Then Grandpa would pour the liquid from the pails into an enormous pot that was simmering over hot coals in the sugar shack. After a few days, the sap was boiled down enough to be the most magical maple syrup anyone has ever tasted. Store-bought has never, ever tasted like the maple syrup my grandpa made.

I don't know how I didn't recognize the building before! I needed to ask Connor more about the trees near the building. Connor had said there were buckets, tools, and glass jars in the basement, but I didn't really think about what they would have been used for until that night, watching my baby sleep. I felt that if this building could be preserved, I could be alright too.

23

THE HAM OPERATOR

Connor Jackson

Katie was getting really antsy and feeling like herself again, closer to her normal, with more energy. She took walks around the floor more often. She had fewer visitors this week than she'd had during the weekend, but new photos, cards, and balloons continued to materialize. Her numbers were still rising, but her white blood cell count was still too low for her to be allowed back on the outside.

After she shared her realization that the building was formerly a sugar shack, I described the tools and metal things we'd found, and she said they sounded like what her family had used to make maple syrup. There were a lot of maple trees around, but I didn't know which species. It made a lot of sense, and I texted the news to Leah, Levi, and Erin when I had the chance. Katie also said that she'd found the information on the triangles in some pretty solid historical journals, but nothing specifically related to the Underground Railroad. Regardless, Leah and I both thought the crusty blankets that were in the basement could be evidence for the shack having been a station.

Leah had done her part of our homework, but there were no big revelations there. The entire park system had been established in 1918 with the acquisition of one plot of land in a nearby town. (When she told us that, we realized that the Park District had recently celebrated their hundredth anniversary.) The property that contained our building and some of the trail had been bought in the 1930s. None of the trails were initially paved with blacktop but were either just dirt, stones, or crushed rock.

———

AFTER WORK, I stopped at a store to get the beer and headed to Richard's house to learn what a huge antenna like the one next to the building might do. He lived in a well-kept yellow house with what I recognized as an old, three-sided TV antenna tower strapped to its side. The tower was connected to the house by thick guyed wires. Like our building's antenna, it was taller than all the telephone and electrical poles in the neighborhood.

I knocked on the front door and Richard immediately answered, as if he had been waiting for me.

"Well, hello! You must be Connor. And with an offering of beer! Come on in with that!" Richard looked older than Claire. He was thin and had a close-cropped gray beard and mustache.

Richard's wife also came to the foyer to say hello. Her

name was Mary, and she was petite, coming just to my shoulder. Like Claire, she also offered cookies. My clean eating was not going well this week!

"So you're here to talk about the antenna on the trail behind your condo complex?" Richard asked as we settled into his den. The equipment held in glass cabinets and shelves above the desk distracted me.

"Yeah, Claire tells me you know about this sort of thing." I gestured at the shelves. "Is all this stuff for HAM radios?" I asked, my eyes unable to land on any one item. There were so many switches and dials.

"It sure is. I've been a HAM operator since I was in high school. Back then, I didn't have as much equipment, of course. I run a website called Happy HAMs where I help people get ready for their license tests, too. By day, I'm a fisheries biologist for the state."

"Not very related, are they: fish and, uh, radio?" My awkwardness was already seeping out.

"Well, they're actually a bit of opposites. Fish are in rivers and lakes, in the valleys. We live on one of the highest hills in the county. Did you see my antenna outside?" I nodded. "We're at the top of the watershed so that I can get my antenna really high, the opposite of the fish at the bottom!"

"I like it. So you're either at the highest point or the lowest point of the watershed." I remembered from college biology that a watershed was the land around a body of water whose surface and groundwater was connected to that body of water.

"Have you ever worked a HAM radio before?" Richard asked me.

"No, I haven't. Judging from your collection, there's a lot to take in," I said.

"Well, let me show you how to do it!" It turned out that most of the equipment in his den helped to broadcast his signal further. He could have used just a modern handheld device if he had wanted, but Richard liked the nostalgic challenge of using gear that had been made before he was born. We donned headphones and spoke into an old microphone that stood on the desk. As we worked the equipment, Richard gave me a bit of a history lesson. I didn't realize that HAM radios were invented in the late 1800s and that signals actually bounced off the moon. Richard showed me his station log, the list of contacts he'd made, and his broadcasts. He told me he often listened to police communication channels and admitted that he'd heard about the break-in last Thursday. So many more people knew about it than I'd ever imagined!

"So about that building..." I led Richard into a conversation about the reason I was really there.

"Yeah, that little brick building with the antenna behind your condo complex?" Richard took off his headphones so we could talk more directly, and I copied him.

"Claire said that you would know about it. But I'm not really connecting the dots beyond the antenna."

"The building was used to house equipment a lot like mine here. The antenna, just like mine too."

"It has a wooden pole, though," I said.

"Oh sure, that doesn't matter. You just have to get high enough to get the signals. That antenna was used as a repeater station for the Park District police force starting back in the fifties."

"The Park District police force. That's cool." I let this information sink in for a beat. "But how did you know it was theirs?"

"Well, I used to listen in with my radio! You can tell how far away a signal is."

"Ok. But why did they need a repeater station?" I asked.

"They just had a hard time communicating over farther distances when the park was expanding and some of their force were patrolling in one valley with other cars in a different valley. You know, in different watersheds."

"Yeah, different watersheds." I smiled.

"So they needed a repeater station to make the broadcast transmit farther. I think that little building was already there and in the perfect spot, so they just retrofitted it."

"That makes sense. But Claire told me it got hit by lightning?"

"I believe that was back in 2007. That was quite a show! I happened to be listening in at the time. I can look in my logs if you're interested in an exact date."

"Oh, no, that's okay. But why did they stop using it . . . or not fix it?"

"The Park District police force uses better equipment nowadays, higher frequencies. They didn't need it anymore. Some of my equipment won't pick up what they use now." I nodded. Our little square of bricks used to help keep people safe in the park, too.

Richard and I chatted for a few more minutes. I was

there less than an hour and thanked him for the lesson on radio signals and antenna.

———

LATER THAT DAY, I mulled over all this new information while running my three easy miles on my normal route by the building. Somehow, I hadn't been past it since the night Leah and I had broken in and attracted the police there. I slowed as I crested the hill. I allowed myself to walk past it to get a good look. Yellow-and-black-striped safety tape had been wound back and forth, both on the door of the building and the gate of the fence. A NO TRESPASSING sign was zip-tied to the side of the fence facing the trail. I surprised myself by feeling proud of causing such a ruckus. I noticed that this pole also had guyed wires like Richard's holding the pole in place. For some reason, they hadn't really registered with me before.

Because of the building, I was distracted during the entire run and didn't get the mile split times I should have. I wasn't happy about this, worrying that I was slowing before the race.

Over the few days I kept thinking of retrieving my lost crowbar, now in the basement, but I didn't dare sneak back into the building after our tangle with the police. I decided it was okay to sacrifice it to the cause. Knowing so many more details about the little building made it feel really important, a part of history.

24

THE PAPER HORNS

Katie Brandt

Finally, my doctor pronounced me well enough to get my stem cells back. I felt much more myself —although tired, always so tired.

Like my last dose of chemo, it didn't feel super-exciting. It felt normal: another injection of fluid being pumped into my body via my neck port. That's what I did all the time. My mom and dad came to hang out for the day, and Travis was on the phone when Connor started the injection. He said he wanted to be there as best he could for this milestone. It would take two hours, and Connor would be in and out to make sure everything went as expected. Connor finished taking my vitals, and my mom took a picture of Connor and me as he was putting it in the port, another milestone photo.

And then suddenly, my parents were blowing those paper horns you give out at kids' birthday parties and throwing pink confetti around.

"What are you doing?" I laughed at them. Connor was laughing, too.

"Celebrating! Your stem cells are going back into your body and cancer is out!" my mom announced, handing both Connor and me horns. My dad kept tooting on his horn for good measure.

"Wait! Do you have a horn too, Travis?" I asked into the phone, hearing more horns going off than just my dad's. He'd taken his phone into the break room at work.

"Sure do!" he said and tooted his horn three times to prove it. "Your mom dropped it off yesterday for me! Time to celebrate, babe!"

"You guys are the best!" I said as Connor honked his horn. A housekeeping person (I think his name was Brandon) poked his head into the room to see what was going on, and my mom actually handed him a horn, too!

"It's so interesting that the room smells like corn," my mom noted as they were picking up the confetti and Connor was packing up his cart. He stored his horn in the pocket of his scrubs.

"Right! I guess it comes from some of the ingredients in the chemo drugs. It is really an unexpected smell," Connor agreed with her. "Just like unexpected horns and confetti," he said with a smile and left my room so we could celebrate on our own.

25

THE LETTER TO THE EDITOR

Connor Jackson

Katie was feeling even better and really pushing the attending physician to let her go early. She wanted to get home to her babies, but we needed to make sure she was healthy enough.

No one was sure where to go next with our research. While nothing was really happening with our building, I worried about how fast the Park District might tear it down under our noses.

I waited with Erin, Clover, and my mom to pick Juney up at the bus stop on her first day of school as a surprise. (What a perk of getting off my nursing shift at three!) She was thrilled that we were all there.

Juney and I did our three-mile loop around the neighborhood. She gave me a deeper first-day-of-school report via purple-glitter bike. Apparently, the day had started out with some tears because her BFF was in another class. She'd known this going in, but it was harder than she thought. Her teacher was so nice, though, that she had a positive day overall. The upgraded jungle gym on the playground was a pretty enormous deal for all the elementary kids. Gram Gram bought all of us some ice cream before dinner as a first-day-of-school treat, as any amazing grandma would. I had remembered to bring the next Lego bag, and I'd also brought a small Duplo set for Clover, who would be back at her school/ day care the next day.

Then Levi grilled chicken for a new tikka masala recipe, and I was in heaven. I did all the dishes and scrubbed the sink as a thank you.

As I was finishing up, Erin came in and put her hand on my back. "Bad news," she said, holding up the local newspaper. I didn't remember that they even got the newspaper.

I wiped my hands on a towel and took it from her. "What's the bad news?"

She pointed to the Letters to the Editor section. I scanned it and latched onto the second letter down. Someone, whoever G.H. was, had written to the editor saying that the "small brick structure along the Park District trail in Hawthorn Heights" was a hazard to the community. Apparently, they'd read the same police report Claire had and were now concerned that "local hoodlums" would use it as a drug-dealing base of operations since the building had been broken into. The person was calling on the Hawthorn Heights mayor to tear down the building.

"Why would anyone say or think these things? Why

would the newspaper even print this?" I said, heat rising in my chest. My voice was louder than I expected it to be.

I looked up and saw Levi leaning against the doorjamb, hands in his pants pockets, shaking his head. "Whoever wrote it really got right on getting their two cents into the newspaper. Sent in their letter right away after learning about the break-in," he said.

"It's a dumb reaction," Erin said. "Let G.H. complain and have their stupid toddler tantrum. Nothing will come of this, Connor. Don't worry about it. They mayor can't do anything like that." She took the newspaper, folded it up, and put it into the recycling bin with a lot more flourish than the action needed.

26

THE DECK CONVERSATION

Connor Jackson

The next day, I went to our local high school track to run mile repeats, which is my favorite sort of training exercise. It really wears me out, so I rarely do it on my own without a training plan to push me. I ran a slow first mile: four laps. Then I really kicked it for a mile, pushing hard. Then a slow half mile and another fast mile. Those first few miles felt great, easy, even. I repeated the kicked-up mile and easy half mile four times. The last two miles were harder, and by the end I was dead. The plan was to run another easy mile after the last fast one, but I just walked. I had no more energy. Again, I worried that I wouldn't make it through the full thirteen in just a few days' time.

Leah and I had planned to get together for a walk after my workout, but I texted and said I didn't think I could move anymore. We settled on beer on her deck, which sounded even better to me.

It was the first time I had been to Leah's place, and her decor was less girly than I expected. And she was wearing her hair down for the first time since I'd met her. That relaxed look on her was really pretty. I took off my running shoes at the door and felt comfortable right away. Her kitten welcomed me by climbing up my leg.

"So how's the researcher-patient?" she asked after we were settled on the deck.

"Doing great. I mean, I can't tell you anything specific. HIPAA and all." She rolled her eyes but made a noise that sounded like agreement. "She's on her way out soon, though, and I'll be able to get her cell phone number and add her to our group text. I'm really going to miss Katie. No one else has ever decorated their room so much or passed out candy. She's got such hope and courage. Not a patient anyone on our floor will forget."

"I'd definitely love to get pictures of those sweet baby girls!"

"For sure. For sure." We were sitting at a table under an umbrella. I took a swig of beer and put my feet up on the wicker chair next to Leah's. We talked a bit about the letter to the editor that had been on my mind since the day before. Like Erin and Levi, she waved it off. Why was I the only one who was nervous about the negative public conversation about my own actions?

"So I've been thinking about the map," she said, as if she were completely changing the subject.

"Yeah, I don't know what to do next."

"I think we should get someone to look at who is an authority on the time period. Or an Underground Railroad historian."

"Yeah. That sounds good. Do you, like, know where to find one?" I asked.

"There's the American Underground Railroad History Museum and Research Center in Toledo."

"Well, you really *have* done your homework. That name wouldn't just flow off my tongue like that." Leah threw her coaster at me, and I dodged, moving my feet, but she motioned for me to put them back. My sweaty, stinky feet—she didn't mind that they were right next to her. I felt embarrassed suddenly that they were so close to her. The fact that she didn't mind was reassuring: she must actually like me.

"I filled out their contact form online, saying that I —*we*—have a map that we'd like to know more about and the person who responded said they'd be happy to look at it."

"That's awesome!"

"I looked up directions, and it's about three hours away," she said.

"So it'd be a bit of a trek. How do we transport the map? Did they have any ideas?"

"I emailed back and forth with a guy who said to put it in a huge Ziploc bag. The kind you'd get in the storage section of the store, not the food section. And then tape the bag to your cookie sheet."

"Okay, sounds simple enough. Well-contained, safe," I said, with picture of this storage system in my head.

"And if we have any of those silica packs that come in packaging, he said to put one or two in the bag with it. But not to keep it like this long term."

"Yeah, that makes sense, too. But when can we go?

I'm busy with the girls on Saturday. Maybe Sunday? I'd need to check my calendar to see which day off I have during the week next week." And as the word "Sunday" came out of my mouth, I considered how I would squeeze in an eleven-mile run, my last long run before the race, before a six-hour car ride.

"Oh, right. The sleepover. And there's some golf involved, I understand?" Leah turned on her teasing voice at the mention of golf.

"Well, putt-putting. No driving ranges!"

"I could help everyone get under par if you're interested in me tagging along." Leah leaned back in her chair.

"I'm sure they'd love to hang out with you, too. I'll clear it with Juney first, though. She's the boss." Leah nodded.

"You're a sweet uncle. But I gotta say, I'm not so sure that the researchers are at the Underground Railroad museum on a Sunday, so we may need to go on a week-day. I can ask. I can also get a weekday off once in a while since the season is winding down. When's your next weekday off?"

"Let me take a look," I said, letting out a breath I didn't realize I was holding with worry about having to skip my run. After a minute on my calendar app, I announced: "I have next Wednesday off. And the following Wednesday I need to *take off* for the court date."

"Right. I need to clear that court date with my boss, too. Not that I'll be telling him what I'd be doing."

"Me, neither," I agreed. "But you think you could get this coming Wednesday off?"

"I do! I'll ask tomorrow."

"Six hours trapped in a car with me might really test how much more you want to hang out with me."

"Trial by fire!" she agreed.

27

THE LAST DAY

Katie Brandt

F inally, my last day in the hospital arrived. As usual, I hardly slept the night before, but it wasn't for the same reasons. I was just too excited! I didn't feel ready physically, but emotionally, I was so done with treating cancer. It was time to be home with my hubby, my babies, my dog, and my own bed. My own bed would be amazing . . . And some actual food—I wanted my hometown pizza so bad! I kept picturing my favorite mug and could almost taste my coffee just the way I liked it as I sipped it at my own kitchen table. I was going to be healthy—for me. I was so ready to be home!

When I woke up, I didn't understand why there seemed to be dog hair in my mouth. Then I realized it was my hair. It was all over the pillow and the floor. I kind of ignored it, let it just sit there, and got into the shower. If I pretended my hair hadn't fallen out overnight, surely it hadn't actually happened.

Travis began texting me early in the morning about his progress: when the kids woke up, when he dropped them off, that he was parked at the hospital. It was putting me back in mom mode a bit, which was good, thinking about the logistics he'd navigated that morning. I'd gotten out of bed by 6:00 a.m., excited but also terrified. Mom mode was scary when you're this tired. But I was scared too - because my hair was finally falling out, and I couldn't help but focus on it as hard as I was trying to ignore it.

I have big, curly hair. Everyone on my mom's side of the family has curls. It's part of my identity. I knew that cancer patients usually went bald and that I needed to expect that as part of the treatment. I had my hairdresser cut a foot and a half off my length months and months ago in anticipation of losing it all. But it was still present, somehow, and I was not bald after eleven rounds of easy pregnancy chemo and then a week straight of the hard stuff there at the hospital. This last day, it finally gave up, and I still wasn't ready.

It came out in tufts in the shower, and there was just no pretending it wasn't happening. I started crying. I was supposed to be so happy, ecstatic to be leaving. But my hair! Today was meant to be wonderful, so losing my hair bothered me that much more. I had to throw gobs of it in the trash can because it was clogging up the drain.

I finished washing and crying in the shower and put my loosening hair up in a towel. I dressed, put on my makeup, and started packing. When I texted my mom and sisters pictures of the clumps of hair, they commiserated with me. They, too, have the curls. To distract myself, I finished taking down everything from the walls. I asked my sweet morning housekeeping lady, Helen, for a few trash bags and put my towels, quilts, blankets, and pillows in those. I folded all my clothes and stuffed them into suitcases with my books, then packed up my snacks and the candy bowl for my caregivers. The candy went on the counter for them to discover later. My brother-in-law had already taken his gaming system home. After packing the dry-erase markers, I wiped the messages the window and then just wiped down every surface. At this point, I was just trying to keep busy. Travis texted that he had parked and was headed my way, but the walk across the hospital still took some time. I couldn't leave the hospital with my hair in a towel. It was time to face it.

And so I took off the towel and looked in the bathroom mirror. I could see patches of my scalp. Some locks were shorter than others, apparently broken. It was a sad sight. I thought, *This is the cost I paid to win the fight; this is what the victor looks like after cancer beats the crap out of her.* And my mascara was running all over my face. It was okay. I may have been bullied beyond recognition, but I was still myself. And today, I was going home, with or without hair.

I called for Zofia, the night nurse, and asked for a comb. I don't have a comb at my house and certainly didn't bring one with me. You don't comb curly hair. She came in and knew I was in a hard place.

"Oh, sweetie, your hair," was all she said. She hugged me before handing over the tool and stood there as I combed my hair in the mirror. With every stroke, I had to clean off the bristles. Zofia took the hair clumps from me as I took them off the comb and held the curls in her hands. An odd thing for her to do, but also very kind and understanding. The combing didn't take long, and when it was over, my hair looked slightly better, managed, at least. I put a little bit of product in it where a few locks still hung on. Zofia left without saying anything and returned with a baggie containing my curls. I hugged her and knew I wouldn't forget her kindness.

———

Connor Jackson

I WAS STILL sore from my track workout when I went running with Eduardo at five the following morning. He was working the late shift, and this was the only time we could squeeze in our weekly three-mile running meeting. I finally told him the story about the building and meeting Leah. He was impressed that I was brave enough to break into an abandoned building. This took me aback. Apparently, I didn't know I had such a reputation for being a rule follower.

On this sore leg day, Katie was soaring in another respect: we would discharge her. On my drive to work, I felt sad to see her go but so happy for her at the same time.

Travis, Katie's husband, showed up right when I arrived at work. We actually rode up in the elevator together. He's one crazy tall guy. And he was ready to get his wife back – he was taking the entire following month off of work to care for her and their brood of kiddos.

When he and I found Katie, she was emotional after waking up to hair all over her pillow. She was ready to let it go and move on, but not without a few tears. I quickly took her morning vitals and then located our hair trimmer. Not all hospital nursing stations stock a hair trimmer. Cancer wards need to have unusual little tools like this in their stash of supplies. I handed it to Travis.

"Yeah. I'll be the one to do it. Are you ready, baby?" Travis asked her, tilting her face up to look into her eyes. This simple statement and the look they exchanged spoke of a relationship like the one Levi and Erin shared. One-half of the couple was brave enough to share their reserve of strength. Travis gave Katie the strength she needed that day. Every patient that left our floor was scared and not feeling totally healthy. They were so excited to be discharged but unsure of the future. They needed to lean on someone, and that day Katie was leaning hard on Travis.

Travis shaved Katie's head in front of a large audience of people on our floor, including nurses, nurses' aides, housekeeping, a social worker, and even the craft cart lady. I wasn't the only one who shed a tear. One of the nurses took a lot of pictures for them, and we posted one on our break room bulletin board.

And so Katie's thick locks became another sacrifice made for her cancer treatment, left behind at the hospital. Before Katie left, we exchanged phone numbers and a long hug.

She and Travis moved all of her stuff to his truck - the pink quilt, pajamas, books, photos, holiday lights, balloons and all of it - feeling lighter than they had since the previous November when they got back the cancer results. She had been scheduled to stay on the stem cell replacement ward for twenty-one days and left on day nineteen. She faced cancer and spat in its face.

I felt moody and mournful the rest of the day, and even my leftover tikka masala for lunch didn't cheer me up. It was like my best friend had moved to a different town.

28

THE SPINNING CLASS

Connor Jackson

After I got home that night, Juney and I video-chatted for a few minutes about our plans for Saturday and confirmed her ice cream flavor request. And she didn't really want Spinning Leah going with us putt-putting. I understood how she felt, seeing that these were *our* plans that hadn't involved Leah from the beginning. When I called Leah to let her know, she was much more disappointed than I thought she'd be.

"What? June doesn't want me to go putt-putting? I mean, why not?"

"Well, I think that she just wants to hang out with me and her sister. I can't blame her for that," I said, really not wanting this to blow up. Why was Leah acting this way? I had certainly never heard this tone from her before.

"But I'm a golfer. I can help everyone do better *golfing.*"

"Oh, I don't doubt that," I assured her. "I just don't

think we're all about being amazing at putt-putting. The girls just want to hang out, and it'll be fun to be bad at it together. It'll be funny. Kids like funny." I was babbling, searching for what to say.

"I don't like breaking plans. I was looking forward to seeing you and hanging out with these other ladies in your life."

"Right, right. But aren't we doing the spinning thing in the morning already? I'm not breaking those plans. And I mean, you kind of invited yourself to a thing that I already had going with Juney and Clover. They're a big deal to me, and if they want to hang out with only me, I'm fine with that. We planned this the day I met you, before we knew each other."

"Well, I thought I was kind of a big deal to you, too."

That really took me aback. Leah was acting like a different person, so defensive and argumentative, and I just didn't know how to react. This always seems to happen with me and the ladies. "Okay. That's cool. Yeah, a big deal sounds right. I really do like you and being with you. But if Juney invited herself to beers on your deck, it would have been a whole different thing than it was last night. You being at Juney's sleepover would give it a different vibe."

"I can be funny. I won't ruin any vibe."

"Oh, sure. I know you're funny. But we're just going to keep it the three of us."

"We?"

I continued without pausing. "I'll see you at spinning, and we'll do the museum next week. We've got the building to figure out. Aren't we part of a team or something? Putt-putting isn't *really* golf." She made a noise of agreement at this. "It's not like they don't like *you*. It's not like *I* don't like you. I want to see you a lot. Just not tomorrow afternoon, when I already have plans to *not* go golfing. To just suck at putt-putting with some cute kids." This somehow diffused the tension.

"Okay. I just really don't like breaking plans."

"Okay. Well, then, let's not make plans I'm not sure I can keep from now on. Like, I am totally planning on sucking at spinning tomorrow too. Lots of sucking at sports I don't do often tomorrow," I said with a laugh.

"You'll be cute while you suck at spinning, though." I could hear her smile. We confirmed where to meet in the morning and got off the phone. She called me cute!

Whew. Note taken: don't make plans I can't keep and leave no doubt that she's a big deal. Relationships were so hard. Maybe it would easier to hang out with my cat roommate and my nieces and never talk to a girl again?

———

I WASN'T SO sure what spinning was all about to begin with. People riding stationary bikes with crazy music?

I met Leah in the entrance to the spinning studio. Erin was standing next to her, looking at her phone. I wasn't expecting Erin. Was Leah trying to make a point of inviting people to things? I didn't know what to think.

"Hi, ladies." I said and kissed them both on the cheek, which was a little weird. Leah seemed happy to see me, no cold shoulder or anything.

"Are you ready to get your butt handed to you?" Erin

asked me, sliding her phone into the pocket of her leggings.

"Well, I haven't been on a bike in a few years beyond a few minutes at the gym, so I'm expecting my butt to hurt no matter what!" I answered, smiling. Erin is competitive. I knew she was looking forward to beating me. Maybe she invited herself?

I had to rent shoes that clipped into the bike pedals. Both Erin and Leah had shoes of their own. Maybe it was like renting bowling shoes at the bowling alley. I tried not to be grossed out by wearing used, formerly sweaty shoes.

"Are you going to wear that baseball cap?" Leah asked as I was putting them on.

"Well, I've been needing something to keep my hair out of my eyes when I'm working out. I've been wearing a hat for running this week. I tried a headband before, and that didn't really do much."

"Yeah, hair in your face while working out is not fun. Why don't you just pull it back? I've got an extra hair tie."

"I don't really think I'm a man-bun kind of guy."

"Well, you didn't think you were the breaking-and-entering kind of guy either," she said, lowering her voice. Then at her normal volume: "You're already a long-hair kind of guy. That kind of goes with being a man-bun kind of guy. I think man buns are cool. If you wear a hat, you're going to get hot. It gets boiling in there."

She had startled me again. "Well, ah. Yeah. I guess I have been proved wrong lately. I *do* get hot when I'm running. That goes with working out." I stood up and tested out the shoes. "But, ah . . . *you* think a man bun is cool?"

"Totally," she said, smiling and pulled a hair tie off her wrist to give to me.

"I guess I could try it today. But I'm telling you, I've tried everything to avoid this."

"Time to stop avoiding it," she said, with her hands on her hips.

Spinning certainly proved to be a great cross-training workout. The music was loud and upbeat. The lights dimmed and brightened throughout the fifty-minute class, depending on how fast we were supposed to be pedaling. Our rotations per minute—RPM—were on the screen, and mine were below the old guy's in the back. But I did spin the whole time. The instructor kept telling us to "find our own hill" and encouraging us to change the resistance as needed. She wanted us to stay within a range of pedal speed, but I often found myself in the lower numbers. There was a lady a row over in a red shirt who gave up and didn't do the standing parts and slowed beyond what we were supposed to. I wasn't at the very bottom of the leaderboard but was really spent by the end. So, yes, I had my butt handed to me. While sporting a man bun.

Both Erin and Leah were near the top of the leaderboard, leapfrogging each other throughout the class. I expect that was how they became friends. They kept egging each other on to catch the one in front. It was funny, and the rest of the class was chuckling at them and cheering for the leader. They really are both so funny.

And admittedly, the hair tie worked perfectly. If Leah thought the man bun was okay, maybe I could, too. My hair didn't stay up completely, but it was finally out of my face.

After class, Erin left quickly, saying that she still needed to help the girls pack and get ready. They were supposed to be at my house right after lunch. Leah and I stood next to her car and talked for a while.

"Listen, I'm sorry I blew up last night," she said. "I haven't mentioned this before, but I'm divorced." I started to say I was sorry to hear that, or "It's okay," or something, but she talked over me. "It's been more than a year now. I moved back here so we wouldn't be in the same town anymore and so I could be close to family again. He broke plans with me left and right when we started to go downhill. Like, I'd be making dinner for the two of us. He knew I was in the act of cooking. And he'd text and say he'd be home late and already ate. We'd have plans to go to a movie Saturday afternoon, and he'd stay at the gym all day. I was just always expecting him, and he'd never be there—and we were married! He was cheating on me, obviously. Obvious now, at least. With three different women. So, I get that time with June and Chloe is special for the three of you. I don't need to barge in. I'm just sensitive when plans get changed unexpectedly." I gave her a hug.

"I appreciate the backstory. Your tone totally surprised me last night. I'm not a big plans-breaker, so I think we'll be in the clear." I smiled at her, glad to be back on better terms. After we said our goodbyes, I ran into the grocery store to stock up on my popcorn and sugary kid cereal, plus my normal, responsible grown-up food and fat-cat cat food.

29

THE SLEEPOVER

Connor Jackson

When Erin, Levi, Juney, and Clover arrived at my place, Erin whisper-demanded to see the map. After getting the girls settled with a game of checkers overseen by Pumpkin, I led Levi and Erin into the office. The map was there, in the same place I had left it. Every time I'd opened this door since its arrival, I kept expecting it to not be there or to have crumbled into a million pieces. But there it was, still lying on the baking sheet on top of my short filing cabinet. Erin actually pulled a magnifying glass out of her purse as she walked in.

"Oh! You came prepared!" I said.

"You know me!" she answered. She and Levi both took turns with the magnifying glass and looked it up and down. "So the building is on the trail up the hill?" she asked after a few minutes of inspection.

"Yep."

"We're going to go take a look." I didn't know why this surprised me. Obviously, she had been planning to get a better look at the map and the building while they were here, but hadn't mentioned it to me beforehand.

Levi shot me one of his overly charismatic smiles and said, "See you in a few, little bro." They went out the back door without even a word to their kiddos. I had to explain to the girls that they were just going on a walk and not actually leaving without saying goodbye. Erin was really on a mission!

We had played three games of checkers (so everyone had a chance to go against each other), and were almost done with our first game of Trouble before they returned. Levi took over my red Trouble markers while Erin talked to me in the kitchen.

"Leah told me about your trip to Toledo this week. I think it's a fantastic idea to have someone with some authority look at it. I contacted our local historical society, too, and they're interested in seeing some photos of the map."

"Oh, man! That's cool," I said, impressed with her resourcefulness. I didn't even know we had a local historical society.

"They're not experts on the Underground Railroad or anything, like the museum. I don't think they can confirm its authenticity. But they may accept it as an artifact for their collection if they like the photos."

"Yeah. It totally belongs in a museum!" We both chuckled at the Indiana Jones reference. We talked more about bedtime routines and pickup time the next day. Levi went outside and put the booster seats in my car.

Then Erin and Levi left for their kid-free night. The girls and I walked down to the playground, and I realized while trying to get across the monkey bars that my shoulders were sore from spinning. Later, we went putt-putting. None of us was any good, and it was a hilarious time.

I had a great night with the nieces, filled with (as planned) pizza, popcorn, and ice cream. We watched a princess movie and ended the night with me reading an entire chapter out of *Harry Potter and the Goblet of Fire,* when Harry fights the dragon. It was really exciting! They didn't put up much of a fight about going to sleep. Pumpkin cuddled up with Clover on the bottom bunk.

30

THE BAND OF ANGRY VILLAGERS

Connor Jackson

The next morning, I made peanut butter pancakes mixed with protein powder for breakfast, topped berries, while the girls ate their sugar-bomb cereal. They both kept eyeing my pancakes as if I might make them eat cardboard, but I just stayed silent and chuckled to myself. We played hide-and-seek and tag in the backyard after breakfast until Levi arrived, a bit before ten.

When they left, I felt ready for the last long run of my training plan. It was eleven miles, and again I put my hair up in a bun. I felt horrible during the entire run. The stashed water and gel combo helped, but I'd done too hard a workout the day before and the ice cream and pizza weighed me down. I felt sluggish. My mile splits really showed it. Despite such a fun evening and morning with the girls, I felt discouraged and defeated at the end of the run.

I decided I needed an update from Katie while I iced my feet and drank electrolytes. I texted her what Erin had said about the museums and asked how she was feeling. She responded quickly with photos of the twin girls and their six-year-old cousin, which cheered me up. She wasn't feeling great, though. I told her not to expect too much and to lean on her people. She had been scheduled to stay in the hospital, with me, for two more days, after all. Sending her encouragement lifted my spirits; helping people always does. I guess that's why I'm a nurse.

After a late lunch, I went to the big-box store to buy the large storage bags we'd need to move the map. I also bought a new notebook because I wanted to take more notes about what we were learning about the building and the map. Erin's conversation with the historical society gave me an idea.

After a quick nap, Pumpkin and I plopped onto the blue couch with the notebook and my laptop to start some research on what it would take to get the building registered as a historic site. Turns out, the National Park Service protects historic sites in one of two ways, either by designating them as National Historic Landmarks or listing them on the National Register of Historic Places. Neither one gave total protection against destruction by the property owner, and neither was quick. I wrote down the steps involved in each and who I should contact on Monday to figure out which one would be more appropriate. Even if a historic designation wouldn't stop the Park District from tearing down the building, it would at least demonstrate that people thought the building was worth keeping.

———

MONDAY BROUGHT a different patient into Katie's room, Al. This new guy was probably twenty years older than she was, and he brought only one family photo to sit on the windowsill for decoration. The room felt drab without Katie's big personality and bright decor. And like every other patient ever before Katie, Al wore the hospital gowns we gave out. Katie was always fully dressed, which made her seem less like a patient. She was always sitting in the bed, of course, but her everyday clothes made a big difference in how comfortable it was to hang out with her. No matter what, we'd all treat Al with the care and dignity he deserved, but he just felt so different from the room's previous occupant.

I left a voicemail for the National Park Service and decided to send an email later that night since I didn't talk to anyone.

My legs were sore, but I still went to the gym that night to do some laps in the pool. I limited myself to twenty-six laps this time, still keeping the faster-down, slower-up rhythm that I'd done in my last pool workout. And swimming is way better with the proper gear: the nose plug made breathing so much easier, and the swimming cap not only kept my hair out of my face but made me at least feel more aerodynamic. Not that I was wearing a speedo or anything!

As I was getting into my car after my workout, I got a call from Leah. She was just getting off work and was so upset that I had a hard time totally understanding her. She said that the Park District had put the demolition of our building on their maintenance crew's work plan for two weeks from now. We didn't have anywhere near the time we needed to get a historic designation. Apparently, after the Letter to the Editor, a group of people attended the Hawthorn Heights City Council meeting that was held just that morning. How convenient that the meeting was held a few days after the letter had been printed. This band of grumpy Hawthorn Heights residents told the council and the mayor that the building needed to be torn down. If I'd known there even was such a thing as a City Council meeting, I might have attended and stood up for myself when they referred to Leah and me as criminals who broke into the building. And despite Erin's confidence that any decision about demolishing the building would take months, they swayed the council members enough to call the Park District executive director that same day. That was not what Erin had promised me. And so now we were up against a deadline and a mob of angry villagers as if we were characters in a video game.

Could we rely on the people at the Underground Railroad museum to help halt action? We didn't even know what they had to say yet. This put me into a major angry worry spiral. I had to sit in my car for several minutes before I drove away. As I was sitting there, Leah sent a group text, and Katie jumped into action right away.

LEAH : OMG! I just heard that the Park Dist is moving ahead with building demo! Slated for 2 wks away!

Erin: No way! This is not cool!

Levi: Crap! What do we do?

Leah: A group of people complained at the city council mtg about it.

Katie: This is SO not cool! I don't even get why they want to tear it down! I'm making a phone call.

Levi: Who you gonna call?

Erin: (Ghostbusters! But not a time for jokes!) This is bad!

Connor: We really don't have time to get the historical stuff ready to stop them at all.

Katie: Who is in charge of this demo project, L? Who should I ask for at admin office?

Leah: Maintenance supervisor, Ralph.

Katie: Calling now.

Connor: Katie, you're awesome!

31

THE MAINTENANCE SUPERVISOR

Katie Brandt

Being at home was awesome. Being surrounded by my family, in my own house, instead of having wires and beeping machines on all sides of me in a sterile hospital room, lifted my spirits and made my body feel like itself again, although weak. When I got the texts from our building mystery team that the Park District had slated the structure for demolition, I was giving Josie a bottle. I knew I had to do something. Fast. Thankfully, my sister Kora was there with me and Travis.

For some reason, I had saved all the numbers I had called to inquire about the building in my phone, so I didn't even have to do a web search for the Park District Administration Office. Tammy answered, as she had last time, but I knew to ask for Ralph and she didn't stall me. When I was on the phone with my target, I went straight into the looking for a lifesaver mode.

"Ralph! This is Katie. I'm in Hawthorn Heights and

just heard that the Park District is tearing down the charming little building on my running route." I was always pretending to live in Connor's town.

"Oh. Yes. I believe that's on our schedule. I don't know the building myself. But, Katie, how did you get this number? I don't usually field calls from the general public."

"I know you're the guy in charge of this, Ralph, and I need a hero," I told him quickly.

"Well, I am a fan of Superman, but I'm not so sure that anyone at the Park District is a hero!" he laughed.

"This little building has a lot of historical significance. We believe it was used by the Underground Railroad as a safe route back in the day. There's a team working to make it a national historic site, and this stuff takes some time. I know that a group of people attended a village council meeting and spurred the council and mayor to contact the Park District, but none of them have the full story. It can't be torn down yet. We need more time."

"Oh, that does sound like a conflict. And that building sounds important." My flattery and uptalking had worked. "Let me pull up some files." I thanked him and heard typing, and then he said, "Listen, it's on the schedule, but I'm the one in charge of the schedule."

"You are? I'm so glad I got you on the phone!" I told him with as much energy as I could muster.

"Yeah. I decide when our equipment moves around the parks. I put that demo on the schedule that day so we could mobilize equipment from a job nearby. Usually, things are on the list for a lot longer."

"So you could change it? Maybe? So we could get

some historical designations ready? Talk to the mayor ourselves?"

"I can change it, but I can't make any promises that it will get off the demo list altogether. I can buy you another month right now." He paused. "Listen, the building's not down yet. The executive director and the board usually make the last call on these sorts of things, and if they learned about the Underground Railroad stuff, they might be able to change her mind. I didn't know. We're not really in the business of tearing down buildings that our communities care about, but if there's another group of people that want it torn down, I can't say. I'm just the scheduling guy."

"The scheduling guy that's saving the day! I knew you were the person to talk to!" I said.

"I'm not making any promises," he cautioned me, "but give me your number. I can at least buy your history team some time."

I told him my number and suggested calling the manager of the golf course that sits right next to the building. He thought he knew who she was. Seed planted. Leah could do the rest, and I could take a nap.

32

THE BALL-GAME DECISION

Connor Jackson

L eah reported that she and Ralph were meeting at the building at ten o'clock Thursday morning. That was good because by then we expected to be armed with new information from the Underground Railroad museum.

I sought out a new trail for my next three-miler. This one was a lot closer to the hospital. It also had a long stretch of exclusively pine forest, which was almost eerie to run through. The race was just a few days away, and I was feeling unprepared, unsure I'd be under my two-hour goal. I didn't feel sluggish at all and did totally hit the mile split times, but the past few runs hadn't been as good. Admittedly, I was happy with my new hair management system. While running, I kept thinking about the village council meeting and the people who wanted our building torn down. It was so disheartening to know that some people had views such different from mine.

That Tuesday night, our dad treated Levi and me to seats right above the dugout for our team's baseball game. Neither of us had been to a game for a few years. Our dad goes pretty often with his buddies and Mom's brother. We agreed to meet at the big mascot statue in front of the ball field.

"There he is!" Dad yelled and waved at me to get my attention in the crowd.

"Hey, Dad!" I yelled back. Levi was right behind, but neither of us had seen each other. We all slapped each other's backs and shook hands.

"Okay, boys, here are your tickets," he told us, handing us each a stub in a very know-it-all yet fatherly way. "Let's get our programs, and I'll show you where our seats are." He led the way without really looking back to make sure we followed.

Our seats had cushions and drink holders—much nicer than any baseball game seat I had occupied before. Levi bought a round of beers before the game started. The thing about ball fields is that they're devoid of anything healthy to eat. During the second inning, Levi and my dad both got huge plastic baseball hats filled with nachos smothered in cheese and jalapeños from a dude walking up and down the aisles. Even without clean-eating aspirations, I would not have wanted to consume so much cheese in one sitting! I excused myself, saying I'd get the next round of beers. I walked up and down the concourse, looking for something I'd want to eat. Somehow, I found a weirdly packaged container of hummus strapped to a bag of carrots at one concession stand. The guy also sold cotton candy, crackerjacks, and nachos with chili on top. I got the hummus-carrot deal, a box of popcorn, and the next round of beers.

As I was passing out the aluminum bottles, Levi winked at me, and I knew I was in trouble. "Has Connor told you he's seeing a new lady?" he asked Dad with a huge smile.

"Oh! No, he hasn't! It's been a while since you've had a steady girl, Connor." It really had. I couldn't even count the number of first dates I'd been on in the past few years.

"Yeah. Her name is Leah," I said. Usually, I'd get all red in the face and stammer. Levi knew how to embarrass me. But no blushing this time. I told him straight. "She's actually a friend of Erin's, and I met her at Clover's party. You probably saw her there, too."

"Well, any friend of Erin's has to be a good girl," Dad said. From a man of few words, this acceptance meant a lot. He wasn't a fan of my last long-term girlfriend, Flora. I had always tried too hard to make her happy, and she had never been supportive of my devotion to running.

"She's great. She's the manager of the Peregrine Falcon Golf Club. I'm spending the day with her tomorrow. We have a lot of fun together." As I said this, it occurred to me that while I had been seeing Leah a lot, Levi was making it sound a lot more serious than either of us had really agreed to.

"Good news. This is good," Dad said, with his eyes back on the pitcher's mound and not on me. That was all the information he needed to know. I knew my mom would probably call me the next day to get a lot more details after he told her about it. I decided then that I was ready to make the relationship as serious as Levi had in mind.

We discussed nothing else as embarrassing or personal for the rest of the night. Our dad is a man of few words but loves to hang out with everyone in our family. Our team won the game, and he was quietly elated.

33

THE WOMAN

Connor Jackson

I ran three miles at 5:15 a.m. at the rec center. My legs were used to afternoon running and were never really happy moving so fast that early in the morning. I ran on the treadmill with earbuds playing an upbeat list. It sucked, but the miles were logged, leaving me with a proud feeling of not cheating on my training plan. I really had stuck to it well.

I admit that I was nervous about leaving the map in my trunk while I was in the rec center, but I knew it would be safe from prying eyes there. Still, I rushed through my shower.

Leah met me in the parking lot, as planned. We left in my car at 6:15 a.m. to make sure we were on time for our 9:30 a.m. appointment with the museum researcher and went through a drive-through to get some coffee before getting on the highway. I had some Sherlock Holmes audiobooks queued up, and Leah was game to listen. I meant to ask her what she wanted to listen to during our road trip, but we never ended up talking about it. Holmes and Watson's adventures hold up really well more than a century later. Although I've read them all, there are so many that are still new on the second or third read or listen. This audiobook had twelve, each about an hour long. We listened to the first one, sipping coffee and pausing every ten minutes or so to discuss how the story was unfolding. I liked to see Leah digging Sherlock! Apparently, she had never read anything beyond one or two of the shorter mysteries in high school.

We listened to "A Scandal in Bohemia," in which Irene Adler outsmarted Sherlock—and he was not happy. He solved the case, but she got away. I paused the player before it went to the next mystery and went bold.

"So, Irene is a pretty big deal to Holmes."

Leah looked at me and smiled at the mention of "pretty big deal," as that was the term we'd kept using in our argument the previous week. "She seems like a *pretty big deal*, being able to outsmart both Sherlock and the Prince of Bohemia."

"Holmes mentions her a lot in future stories, calls her 'The Woman.' Few people knew what he's going to do before he did it—but she did."

"Yeah?" she asked, raising her eyebrows.

"Sherlock isn't interested in her romantically. He's a rare asexual guy with no interest in the ladies."

"He does seem very focused on his work." She was using her teasing voice, unsure where I was going in this conversation.

"And his violin and drugs sometimes," I said.

"Drugs!?" Teasing voice off.

"Well, we haven't gotten to that part yet. But that's not my point. Irene was a big deal to Holmes—and, well, you are a big deal to me," I blurted out.

"A big deal," she repeated. I wasn't sure if she was making fun of me or just agreeing.

"And I think we should define our relationship. We've seen a lot of each other the past few weeks. Done some crazy stuff. I'm including a spinning class, here." She laughed. "So I guess what I'm saying is . . . well, I'm going to call me your girlfriend." I couldn't look at her. I didn't want to *ask* her to be my girlfriend. I wanted to tell her that's what she was to me. It felt right.

"Connor. How about you call me your girlfriend? And I'll call you my boyfriend. I'm the girl here."

"Wait. What?"

"You were asking to call *yourself* my girlfriend."

"Well, I was telling you . . . and I totally meant it the other way around. I mean, of course I did." This wasn't how I wanted the conversation to go. How could I have gotten that wrong?

"Oh, I know! It's a hard question to ask! Well, I am happy with you calling me your girlfriend. We're officially a couple as of"—she made a show of looking at the dashboard clock—"7:37 this morning." She leaned over and kissed me on the cheek.

"So it's official." I smiled.

"So it is. Ready for the next Sherlock?" she asked, turning the conversation on a dime.

"I'm excited for you to hear more Holmes and Watson stories! Totally ready." I unpaused the app, and the first

Sherlock story published, "A Mystery in Scarlet," started. I took a swig of my coffee and took Leah's hand in mine, kissing it before resting our hands between us. It felt good to be an official boyfriend, even if I got laughed at because the ask was so awkward.

34

THE UNDERGROUND RAILROAD
HISTORY MUSEUM

Connor Jackson

The American Underground Railroad History Museum and Research Center was not exactly what I was expecting. It was wider, taking up more space than I thought it would, not tall. I think of museums as tall, solid buildings, but this one was only one story and had a sloping metal roof. It was a dramatic building that I instantly liked.

Our meeting was to be held before the museum opened, so we went to a staff entrance on the side. The researcher, Henry Holbrook, greeted us at the door. He was a tall, graying black man with horn-rimmed glasses. He looked very much the researcher.

"Hello! I'm glad you found us!" Henry said warmly.

I almost said, "Couldn't miss this place!" but Leah was quicker with introductions and thanked him for meeting with us. Henry led us inside, through a hallway lined with framed photos of historical figures and past Executive

Directors of the organization. We settled in a conference room overlooking the city. In the middle of the conference table I set down the tattered, severely creased map inside a storage bag taped to a cookie sheet. It looked pathetic resting there, not so mysterious in the middle of this museum. But when I was fumbling in the dark with police sirens going off, finding it had felt so earth-shattering.

"A very interesting artifact!" Henry exclaimed after I set it down. He held his index finger under his chin, looking the map up and down.

"Well, we were pretty excited to find it!" I told him. He nodded enthusiastically and got down to business.

Henry had printed the emails that he and Leah had exchanged and had them in a manila folder, along with a printed map of where our building was. He asked us to confirm the location on the map where the building was located. He had it right. Then he asked us to fill out some forms and write a description of how and where we found the map. Each of us filled one out.

While we were writing, Henry pulled on white gloves and asked, "May I?" We both nodded and he opened the bag gingerly. Ever so carefully, he laid the map out on a black cloth and stared at it some more. He applied one drop of a clear liquid to a corner and took some notes. He put another corner under a microscope, taking notes as he went. Henry really seemed to know his stuff and took his inspection very seriously.

I finished writing first and went to stand next to Henry. Our "artifact" looked more official under his gaze, on top of the black cloth instead of my cookie sheet.

Henry took some photos and even asked to take a photo of us so he could remember our faces.

"Would you mind if we took a picture of you and your inspection?" Leah asked. I was glad she did. I knew our crew back home all wished they could be here, and a photo of his work would be cool.

"It appears to be genuine," Henry told us after a few more minutes. "The paper is of the time period, as far as I can tell. I agree with your theory of the map being drawn for a person who could not read by a person who could more than likely read themselves. It is a unique artifact. We have nothing like it here."

"That's encouraging," I said, just as Leah asked, "How do you decide if you want it here?" She and I looked at each other and grinned.

"I know you are here from out of town and will be leaving today. I will meet with some colleagues this morning and can give you a preliminary decision after lunchtime."

"That sounds good," I said. "We have another request." Leah nodded.

"What's that?" Henry asked.

"The building where we found the map. The owners are planning on tearing it down."

"That would be very unfortunate," Henry said, looking from me to Leah.

Leah jumped in and spoke quickly. "We were hoping, with your findings, that you could help prove the historical significance of the building for us. It's not just the owners of the building that are unsure of its importance, but some of the community members as well. But they don't know the entire story."

"Certainly, this map was created in the 1800s, and you are saying that the building itself is slated for destruction?" We nodded. He paused to collect his thoughts, index finger rubbing his chin again, while Leah started picking at thumb with her forefinger. "When I meet with my colleagues, I can ask their thoughts on drafting a letter of support to impede the building's destruction. Our support may help your cause, but we certainly can't promise anything."

"Awesome!" I yelled, as Leah jumped up from her chair in excitement.

"I'll plan to meet you in the lobby at one thirty. I've arranged for free admission to the museum for you both. Just tell them your names at the registration desk. We do have a gift shop with snacks, but you'll have to find lunch across the street or downtown. You'll find some suggested restaurants in the brochures at registration, as well."

We said more thank-yous and goodbyes and were led through more administration hallways to the lobby.

———

AFTER CHECKING IN, we walked around, experiencing the exhibits, watching short films without saying much to each other. There were maps showing the routes slaves were thought to have taken from the South to the North. Displays depicted hiding places that runaway slaves would have used at safe houses, along with how they were treated as slaves in the South.

Certainly, I'd learned about the Underground Railroad and slavery in school. I'd watched *Roots* and *Harriet*. But slavery was far more gruesome than my textbooks had shown. People treating other people as commodities, as though they were not fellow humans. The exhibits focusing on slavery in today's world were the hardest for me. They showed that it's actually "cheaper" to buy slaves now than it was in the 1800s.

We checked out the gift shop once we were done at the museum. I have a magnet collection from museums and other places I've visited. But I didn't feel right buying an American Underground Railroad History Museum and Research Center magnet. It wasn't a trophy visit. Instead, I bought a book on modern slavery and left all the cash in my wallet in the donation box. We ate lunch at a cafe across the street that the gift store clerk recommended.

———

HENRY WAS WAITING for us in the lobby when we returned from lunch. His seriousness made him hard to read. Was he about to tell us good news or not? Again, he led us through the building to the conference table where another person was waiting, sitting with the map. Henry introduced us to a woman with tiny dreadlocks and bright pink lipstick, Izla Williams, the director of curation at the museum. Again, Leah started with a polite thank-you for meeting with us. I was learning that Leah was better at navigating formal situations than I was—I just wanted to push into the business.

After the niceties, Izla told us, "We appreciate both of you taking the time out of your work week to meet with us. We are impressed with your specimen and thankful for your careful delivery."

"We're really excited about it!" I blurted out.

"I'm glad you are! It is an exciting discovery. Tell me a bit more about the building where you found it," she requested.

Leah and I took turns describing the structure and the area surrounding it, our sugar shack theories, and our knowledge of how the Park District used it.

"It does appear that the building you're describing is this structure on the map," Izla stated.

"We're here to both learn more about the map's origin and purpose as well as defend the building," Leah told Izla and Henry.

"Yes. I looked in our records and we have no information about your town taking part in the Underground Railroad prior to this map's documentation. I believe that it is a proof of activity there," Henry said, speaking for the first time during our second meeting.

"This is great!" I said.

"It is very exciting to add to the collective history of the Underground Railroad movement," Izla agreed with a big smile. "It's a rare occurrence to discover something new like this."

"Yes, we believe this is an important discovery. We have scanned it and will add both the information about it that you provided and the information contained in it to our archives. We share the archives with other museums, research institutes, and universities worldwide. We have a report of the information I gathered about the paper and what the map depicts that you can provide to your Park District. Here is a copy." He slid a folder across the table toward us. "I will also email you a digital draft. We've also put together a letter to the District and your village council, signed by our Executive Director, requesting that they do not tear down the structure."

"Whoa!" I said at the same time that Leah exclaimed, "We so appreciate this! You're really sticking out your neck for us!"

Izla told us, "As I said, it's not common to find new information such as this. History is easily forgotten and lost. We do stick out our necks for structures with historical significance. We're happy to do it."

Leah and I both were sporting huge smiles.

"In fact, we expect that this will be a bit of a big news story in your region, if not the entire state," Henry told us. "We believe that the Park District and village will find this a point of pride and may want to partner with us on media relations about the news."

"Then they for sure wouldn't tear down the building!" I said.

"I agree," Henry said with a smile.

Izla continued, placing both of her hands on the conference table. "We don't have all good news, I'm sorry to say. The condition of the paper is very degraded and would not make a solid museum piece here. It is unfortunate." Leah and I both made deflated noises, and she paused. "We expect your local historical society or other nearby regional museums would be interested in acquiring it, especially with its new revelations. Or perhaps the village has a small history display in their offices. You are welcome to share our report with any of them, and we can draft a letter of recommendation, as needed."

"Someone else who has been helping us with the research has been talking with the local historical society," Leah said.

"That's good. We'd be happy to help in those conversations in any way," Izla said.

"We really appreciate your study of the map," Leah told both Izla and Henry. "You've helped validate its importance and the building where we found it."

"For sure," I added, dumbly nodding. The meeting ended soon after, and we said our goodbyes.

So we had good news and bad news to share with Levi, Erin, and Katie. The map had been authenticated and we had a letter to give to the Park District, village counsel, and historical society stating the historical importance of the building. But no home for the map other than my office. We placed it back in my trunk and headed up the highway.

35

THE MEETING AT THE BUILDING

Connor Jackson

We said little during the first twenty minutes of the ride. I'm not sure why I didn't start the next Holmes and Watson story, but I was in my head about the museum, our meetings about the map, and my new boyfriend status. It seemed that Leah was good to sit and think as well. We ended up talking a lot more about the museum and listened to only one more story.

We agreed that Leah would call Erin and Levi after they got home from work to tell them the map news and that I'd call Katie. We thought dropping the news should be done over the phone, not texted. Leah and I said our goodbyes in the rec center parking lot. We didn't have any plans for meeting soon, but they were certainly implied.

I wasn't really sure when to call Katie. I thought she'd probably be home all the time, but sleeping a lot. I called soon after getting home, about five thirty.

She answered the phone, exclaiming, "Connor! I didn't expect you to ever actually call me, dude!"

"Well, hello yourself! How are you? How are you feeling?" I started pacing around the living room.

"You're not calling to ask me how I'm feeling!"

"Okay, you got me there. I just thought I should tell you about our findings today at the museum instead of texting. But I still want to know how you're doing!" I told her.

"Are you about to tell me some major bad news, then?"

"Katie! How are you? Tell me that first."

"Well, I'm still pretty tired. I'm napping a lot. My head is super cold. You know, from not having any hair. Been wearing a lot of beanies. It's so good for me to be home, though. My bed feels amazing. Seeing my babies and having Travis here is awesome."

"This sounds good! You're on the mend!" I actually was pumping my free fist in the air. It's rare to get an update from a patient after they leave our floor, and knowing that this particular lady was doing well felt like such a victory.

"Yeah, I think so."

"So, map news." I got right down to business now.

"Tell it to me, man!" And I did. Leah was planning on emailing copies of the letter first thing in the morning to Executive Director Alice Fitzgerald, to Ralph, whom she'd be meeting with that day, and to Warren Ellsworth, her boss. She was hoping for an immediate pause in tearing down the building, even if no actual decision happened for a few weeks. In the meantime, we thought

Erin could convince our local historical society people to ask for the map to be placed in their hands. Katie was enthusiastic about the news, but like Leah and I, discouraged that it was not well preserved enough for the American Underground Railroad History Museum and Research Center.

————

THURSDAY, I was back at work, monitoring Al's progress. He was at the end of the chemo and feeling bad. It's a predictable schedule. He had visitors most days, and lots of his grandkids' art now decorated his walls. No pink comforter or dry-erase messages on the window, though. All morning I was on pins and needles, expecting a text from Leah about her meeting with Ralph.

Finally, just before eleven, Erin texted and asked if I could talk about the building. Why was Erin calling me? Had she already spoken with Leah? I told my fellow nurse that I needed to step out for a few minutes, and she was okay with it.

"Hey, there! What's up? What do you know?" I said when Erin answered the phone. I took the call in one of the small conference rooms we use to confer with families.

"Chloe and I happened to be going on a bike ride past the building when Leah had her meeting with Ralph," she told me in a singsong voice.

"Oh, Erin! You are such a troublemaker! Always have to be the first in the know!"

"I won't deny either of those accusations," she said. I

knew she was smiling by the tone of her voice. "Chloe and I are on the way to the library but before we get there, we figured we should go on a bike ride. We parked at your house to ride on the trail behind your place, of course."

"So what did you find out?!" Again, I was pacing the room, impatient.

"Leah was right on time and told Clover some jokes until Ralph got there. He actually parked his truck right on the trail, in everyone's way. Not a great first impression." I made some annoyed noises to agree with her. "But Leah knew him and was chummy. As you know, she's really great at chatting people up."

"I do. She showed that off yesterday at the museum."

"Right. Leah introduced me and Chloe as her friends —ahem—not her *boyfriend's sister-in-law*. We'll talk about *that* in a minute. I acted as though I really had just happened past at the time and was *ever so interested*. Leah described how the Park District had used the building in the past and then how its historical significance has been discovered. Nothing about *who* had made the discovery. He seemed pretty bored with what she was saying, walking around the fence and looking it up and down as she talked. He didn't really let her finish and then took off the warning tape and went inside. Leah followed. Chloe and I just stood outside. I really wish I could have gotten in! I should have that time Levi and I were there. I just didn't want to end up in such trouble like *you*!"

"Yeah, yeah," I said in response, rolling my eyes and laughing.

"They weren't in there very long. He had a flashlight

with him, so I think he got a good look." I could hear a blinker in the background. "She said he did glance in the trapdoor."

"Okay . . ." I said, wanting to know the conclusion.

"When they came out, Ralph read through the papers Leah brought from the museum and finally seemed impressed!"

"Impressed! Great!" I jumped up and down.

"Yeah. He said that if a national museum with researchers thinks it's important, he couldn't argue. But Ralph doesn't have the final say. He just isn't going to tear it down on the proposed schedule. Leah still needs to hear from her boss, whom she doesn't see regularly at the admin building, and the executive director. When she left the building to walk back to work, she hadn't heard from either of them yet."

"Right, right," I said, wondering how much more convincing the higher-ups would need.

"And, I heard from the local historical society. They're all volunteers, you know, so they are slow to respond. They need some more info from us and would like some of us to attend their next monthly meeting and show them the map."

"That sounds good. Do they want to see the letter from the American Underground Railroad History Museum and Research Center?"

"I don't know that they are aware of that yet. I need to get a copy from Leah," Erin said.

"Yeah, I'm sure that won't be too hard. Text us all the meeting date and I'm sure a couple of us can attend. Maybe not Katie."

"So Leah and you are officially together now? A *couple*." Erin changed the subject quickly while I was still in mid-thought about the meeting.

"Yep! We are! As of yesterday morning." I just owned it. What else was I going to do?

"I like you two together. I'm happy for you, Connor."

"Well, thanks. It's good. I'm happy, too."

"Chloe wants to say hello. I'm going to hand her the phone. We're almost there." And so I talked to Chloe about her bike ride and seeing "Spinning Leah." She told me about the books she was returning to the library. We only talked for a few minutes because I had to get back to work and she was almost at the library.

Soon after that, a flurry of conversation erupted from our group text about the morning's news. I didn't respond much since I had a full patient load that day. Another patient was being discharged, and that occurrence is always a catalyst for an avalanche of record keeping.

That night, I had a five-mile tempo run: three fast miles sandwiched between two slower ones. I ran past the building, feeling excited, finally able to really think about the business with the map. I could tell the tape had been moved around and the plants within the fence were trampled again. The whole time I was running, I was picturing runaway slaves pushing through the woods, following our map to the building. They ran in the same area where I was now, running for their freedom. They would check for trees pictured on the map and the big rocks. I had it so easy on the trail, with no briars or undergrowth to hinder me. I didn't have to look anywhere but down to see where I needed to go, no searching for the next milestone. And no one chasing me, wanting to drag me back to a horrible life of torture and servitude. They were running toward freedom, toward a life they wanted to live for themselves. I was just running for the sake of it. It felt petty and unimportant. I had worked so hard to train for this race, had been obsessive about sticking to the training plan. And suddenly, I was wondering if it was worth the effort at all. With all these doubts and ideas swirling through my head, I ran faster than I should have and beat every mile split I was supposed to.

36

THE DOUBTS

Connor Jackson

Pumpkin Muffin woke me up early the next morning, begging for his breakfast before I wanted to get out of bed. Despite playing a mindless video game after my run the night before, I still hadn't shaken the gloomy feelings caused by thinking about the runaway slaves and my own pointless running.

Work was slower than normal. We didn't have a new patient to fill the newly empty room, so I had one less patient to cover than the other nurses that day. That left me with too much time to be in my head.

Leah and I agreed to talk on my lunch break to figure out plans for a dinner date that night, our first date as a couple. Hearing from her pulled me out of my funk, thankfully. I told her that it was her turn to choose the eatery, and she came up my favorite restaurant, Saffron and Naan, without even knowing it was my place! She loves Indian food, too. I told her that they'd know what I wanted to order before we even sat down. She really liked this idea. She had other news, too.

Her boss had emailed, asking her to come to his office before she even got to work that day. She told me that she was worried that he had finally heard about our run-in with the police and would fire her for being too involved with the building. Dead wrong. Leah was kind of new to the job and didn't know Warren that well. Turned out, he was a huge history buff and was even on our local historical society's board. He was thrilled to get a letter addressed to him from the American Underground Railroad History Museum and Research Center! The existence of the map was new to Warren, and he asked for the opportunity to study it himself. She finally came clean and told him that she had broken into the building with me. He didn't like that but was happy to support us at the upcoming historical society meeting, and possibly a village council meeting, if needed. Warren also asked to meet her at the building that afternoon. She showed him pictures of the map, and he was very enthusiastic. She told him that she could bring it to him on Monday.

———

IT WAS FRIDAY, so I was running with Ed after work. He had an early shift and was waiting for me at our mid-trail meeting spot. He was hanging out at the playground area, alternating between chin-ups on the monkey bars and burpees in the crushed tire playground mulch. I avoid those exercises because they're so hard! He was exercising to pass the time because he's as obsessed with bodybuilding as I am with running. You'd never catch me doing burpees while waiting for anything, that's for sure. I took my time walking over to him from the parking lot, watching him from afar, exercising in the sunshine on playground equipment. It made me appreciate his drive, and I knew I could talk to him about my low feelings about running. These feelings were coming at the exact wrong time, just days before my big race.

I jogged the last one hundred feet to him. We did our usual bro-hug, and right away he asked me about the big stuff: "What's up with the building being torn down? Are you ready for the big race on Sunday?"

I started with updates about the map and building and left the longer conversation I needed to have about the race for later. "Leah and I had a meeting at that museum I was telling you about. They said that the map confirms that our town was involved with the Under- ground Railroad, so it is a pretty big deal."

"Alright! Alright!" he replied, smiling, and we headed toward the trail. I filled him in on the rest of the discov- eries we'd made since I'd last seen him. As we started our pre-run stretches on the grass, I told him about my run the previous night and my sudden feelings about the pettiness of running, and listened intently.

"Aw, man! Petty?" he said, shaking his head. "I mean, I get that you're feeling down on yourself once in a while. Especially before your big race: having jitters and doubts comes with the territory. But exercise isn't petty!"

"But compared to the runaway slaves I've been thinking about so much, my life is too easy."

"Well, white boy, you know you *do* have it easy! Don't

be asking for life to get harder! But my bodybuilding, your running: these aren't insignificant endeavors. They aren't petty. We're healthier for our exercise and don't have to worry as much about heart disease and all the other obesity-related diseases. Exercise is a discipline. It makes us better people: stronger inside and out. Am I right?"

"Yeah. Stronger inside and out. I like that."

"I mean, I'm sure the people who were following the map had their own hobbies, too. Like whittling wood into sculptures of animals or making up songs or—something. I don't know what they did back then! But your hobby is important to *you*. I'm sure what they liked to do was important to them, and that slavery didn't let them do it as much as they wanted. So they ran through the woods toward a life of their own. Freedom to do what *they* wanted, *when* they wanted. America is a place where we are all supposed to be able to do what we want, right?"

"Well, as long as it's legal."

"Oh, sure. So running is your thing, and you're passionate about it. Don't get down on yourself about that. It's not petty." He was done stretching and was really looking me in the eye.

"Yeah. Okay. You're right." He was convincing, but the intense eye contact was making me uncomfortable.

"Your race is going to be awesome. You've put in all the time. All the miles. And it's not supposed to be weirdly windy or cold or anything like that dumb time I tried to run a half-marathon."

"Thanks, Ed. I really needed your pep talk!" After a beat, I added, "It wasn't dumb when you ran a half!"

He pushed me in disagreement, and as I recovered,

we started running. It was a good three miles. And some-how, he didn't say a single thing about my new-normal man bun.

Later I had a great night with Leah, starting at Saffron and Naan. We ordered a few dishes to share, including a lamb meal that I'd never had before. The guy who usually hands me my takeout bag kept shaking his head and smiling to see me eating something different and actually sitting down at a table. Leah and I hung out at my place afterward, watching a Sherlock Holmes movie and spent some time just staring at the map in my office.

———

I HAD to work the Saturday before the big race, which helped to keep my mind on other things. My training plan mandated a rest day from working out. I wore my running shoes to work to give my feet an extra treat.

I had a really hard time deciding what to eat that day. All the advice I had read was to eat my "normal" diet. But what about the whole carb-loading theory? And what's really normal? I knew pizza and ice cream probably weren't the best idea from the week before with the girls.

My mom called during my lunch break and asked if I wanted to come over for dinner that night. She was going to ask Levi's family, too. After hearing about my food predicament, she said she'd make anything I wanted.

"Name it, honey! I won't even give Levi an option. They'll eat anything, anyway."

"I think carb-loading is a tried-and-true pre-race tech-nique. Could we do spaghetti?" I asked.

"Absolutely! Do you want garlic bread too? What about salad?"

"Garlic bread, salad. Yeah, that all sounds great. Could we do meatless? Like those frozen vegetarian meatballs, so I'm not eating some heavy red meat before the race?"

"Yeah. We all like those. Sounds great. I'll have the meal ready by six, but you feel free to show up earlier, honey," she said.

"Thanks, Mom. I appreciate you making a special dinner for me."

"We're all proud of you for training so hard for this. You're going to do great. I know it!"

"Aw, Mom. You're the best. Thanks. See you tonight."

Before going to my parents' house, I needed to pick up my race packet with my bib number and all the freebies and advertisements. That let me scope out the parking situation better in relation to the starting area.

We had a really nice evening. I left at the same time as Levi and his family, because I wanted to go to bed at the same time as Juney and Clover. I would be getting up early and knew I'd have a hard time getting to sleep no matter what time I settled in.

I set out all my clothes, bib number with the safety pins already attached, and a hoodie to wear to the race and leave in the car. Next to the clothes, I even laid out the gel pack and the hair tie Leah gave me. All my stuff was ready. I knew where to park. I was set. There was nothing else to do but sleep, eat, and be on time. If I could do that, I'd be good to go.

37

THE RACE

Connor Jackson

The marathon, half-marathon, and 10K all officially started at 7:00 a.m. I set my alarm for five. Predictably, I had a hard time falling asleep and staying asleep that night. It was good that I went to bed early. I made the breakfast from last weekend: whole wheat pancakes with protein powder and peanut butter. Pumpkin Muffin was bleary-eyed as he watched me prepare my meal. He sat on the counter as I ate and drank some coffee at the bar. I got dressed quickly and was on the road by five thirty.

I parked a few blocks farther away than I needed to, but I wanted to make sure I found a parking spot without circling the area for long. I also didn't have to pay twenty dollars to park. I took off my hoodie and left it in the car. My bib had both my name and my number on it. You can pay an extra dollar for your name, and I thought, why not? As I was walking to the waiting area a few minutes after six, Leah called to wish me luck. It was good to hear her voice. I was feeling really nervous and cold, wishing I hadn't left the hoodie. Then I got a text from Erin with a video that she had obviously taken the night before, with the girls saying, "Good luck, Uncle Connor! We love you!" She told me she was going back to bed but would check in later.

I found a bathroom inside and warmed up. They were handing out coffee and I took a cup, but didn't drink even half of it. I was starting to think that I should have run some of my longer runs this early in the morning. Would my legs be ready to go at this time of day? I did some jumping jacks and stretches to get my body moving. I felt like I was there too early and had nothing to do. I was restless, just walking around through an immense crowd of people. The runners' bibs were different colors depending on the length of their race. The half-marathon bibs were blue. I like blue. Seemed like a good thing.

At 6:40 a.m., Ed called. "You've got this, man! You are ready! And. Running. Is. Important!"

"Thanks for the encouragement!" I yelled into my phone over the din of the crowd. As I was zipping my phone into the pocket with my car key at the small of my back, I got another text from a coworker, and then one from Katie and then my dad. It was a deluge! My people were really showing some love, and it lifted my spirits. I *had* put in the miles. I was cold, but I was ready.

There were volunteer Pace Keepers who held up signs on wooden sticks high above their heads who would run at a specific time per mile. They were wearing yellow vests. I slid in between the nine- and eight-and-a-half-minute-mile paces. When I'm running just a few miles, I go faster, but today, I wanted to play it safe and finish strong. At this pace, I'd be under two hours for sure. I didn't want to push myself too hard. The guy on the loudspeaker was telling people about the Pace Keepers and announcing the number of minutes until the race started. To my left was a woman in a pink shirt with long braid and a yellow bib, showing that she was running the full marathon. She was chatting with a friend on her other side but gave me a nod. I jumped up and down and did some more stretches. The guy on my right side, wearing a blue bib, seemed to like this idea and started jumping too. I felt like I needed to pee again, although I had just gone. It was nerves. I felt my phone buzz again on my back but didn't want to look at it anymore. The race was starting in just a few minutes.

The announcer came on again, thanking the race sponsors and the runners for participating. Then he actually started a countdown, as if we were in a space shuttle lifting off from Earth. Five, four, three, two—and on one, a gun was fired. Everyone shuffled forward a few steps. When you're not in the very front, you have to wait until the crowd moves to really start running. Nothing like a space shuttle liftoff!

After about two minutes the crowd of runners finally spread out, and I could finally stretch my legs out into my stride. I didn't see the woman with the pink shirt and braid at all. Even though it was early, my legs were actually feeling better than I expected, not leaden like as they had on Wednesday during the treadmill miles at 5:15 a.m. There were police motorcycles monitoring our progress and stopping traffic from entering the streets where we were running.

By the first mile marker, I wasn't cold anymore and was feeling just fine. I kept my 8:30 Pace Keeper about one hundred feet in front of me, and that first mile was right on the 8:30 split. The Pace Keeper really knew what he was doing. There was a timekeeper yelling out times with a huge digital clock on a tripod at every mile marker. Right after the first mile marker, I passed a guy wearing a superhero Flash costume. It didn't seem appropriate for a marathon, but running superheroes are cool. I wondered if it made him feel faster. There were other runners in costumes and wacky getups, but Flash made the biggest impact on me.

The route twisted from the commercial downtown starting area into residential neighborhoods. Along these streets, there were families on lawn chairs with blankets on their laps cheering us on, ringing bells, and holding signs. I was surprised how much the little kids' encouragement affected me. The last time I ran such a long race, Clover was just three and Juney was five. They were too small to know what was going on. I think those little kids waving banners took on my nieces' forms to me.

The first drink station was at mile three. I grabbed a cup and took a small swig of water. I finally caught sight of my neighbor in pink with the braid and gave her a little wave, which she returned.

After mile four, the marathoners peeled away onto a different course: the yellow bibs went left, and all the blue bibs stayed to the right, along with me and the red 10K racer bibs. There was a guy standing at the intersection next to the sign to make sure everyone went in the correct color-coded direction.

Just after the seven-mile mark, we took an empty on-ramp onto the closed highway, which was surreal. It was just us blue bib wearers now; the red bibs had split off in the middle of mile four, going in a different direction for a shorter route. Driving an open highway always feels so spacious and free; running an open highway feels even more free. I knew this section of the state route well, and it was such a different view, no car surrounding me, going so much slower. I noticed weeds growing in cracks between the asphalt near the edges and a rabbit on the median. These would have always been there, but I'd always been going faster than sixty-five miles an hour, not eight.

I found the gel in my pocket and slurped it down. Right as I was done with it, there was a commotion ahead. I could see the runners swerving to change directions and realized that there was a person on the ground. As I got closer, I realized it was my jumping buddy from the starting line! I got to him and bent down to ask what was going on and saw right away that his ankle was already swelling.

"Oh, man. I fell. It's bad," he told me through the pain. He was grimacing and holding his hurt leg. I told him I was a nurse and looked around for a police motor-cycle to call for help or one of the rare roving ambulances. As I surveyed the scene, I saw my 8:30 Pace Keeper run down the hill away from us. Nurse mode was kicking in, and I just let the sign go. Someone actually tripped over my friend's outstretched leg before I could respond to him, and he yelled in pain.

"Okay, buddy, we really need to get you out of the road. I don't want you to put any weight on this leg," I said. I put my shoulder under his armpit and helped him stand. We slowly made our way to the right vehicle pull-off zone with runners zigzagging around us.

"Can I help you take off your shoe? I'm sorry to say that you're not going to finish the race," I told him.

"Yeah. There's no way. I can't even stand! I don't think I can bend my knee to get to my shoe. Thanks for your help—but you're losing your pace group!"

"It's okay. Like I said, I'm a nurse. I'll get you settled and I'll catch up." And so I took off his shoe and sock. His ankle was obviously twisted, and he'd really hit his knee on the asphalt, too. I wondered if I should call 911 since I hadn't seen any other help. I wished I had ice and bandages for his bloody knee. I brushed some debris off it and put pressure on the wound with his sock. After a little more than a minute, I looked up to see a blessed motorcycle. The policeman slowed, balancing the bike with his feet, and radioed his location to someone, requesting medical aid with very few words. He was efficient and to the point.

"Get running!" the policeman waved at me. "I'll make sure he's safe. Finish the race!" He was off his motorcycle and slapped me on the back. He didn't have to tell me twice. I stood and patted the injured man's shoulder before pulling back into the crowd.

"Finish strong!" my injured neighbor yelled after me.

And so I ran. The few minutes' reprieve gave me a

major second wind. I was passing people as if I were flying. I felt a bit of a high from helping someone I'd never see again, someone without cancer but who also just had a major setback. This guy would have trained as hard as I had but would not finish this race that we had both been preparing for. I felt for him and was glad I got him to safety. I hoped he'd run again and be okay. I'd finish the race for us both.

Then, somehow, ahead of me was a sign bobbing up and down. The sign read 8:30. I had caught up with my Pace Keeper! I have no idea how I caught him. No idea how the last mile felt like it hadn't happened.

And then, inexplicably, I passed him. My legs were going on autopilot, and I just whizzed right by without looking back. I wondered if running this fast was a good idea. My plan was to play it safe, to stick with this Pace Keeper and even hold back if I had to. But then I thought about Katie and the guy with the twisted ankle. Neither of them would be running any time soon. Katie would be crazy proud of me if I finished faster than I planned to. I felt great. I decided to let my body be my guide, take the risk, and keep up this quick pace. I'd run my last few training runs faster than my plan dictated, after all, and felt confident I could finish strong.

We were only on the highway for another mile or so. I liked running down the highway exit on my feet instead of on the wheels of a car. It was such a different perspective! I also caught up with the man in the Flash costume—and passed him.

By the middle of mile ten, I was feeling tired. My helper's high was gone. The adrenaline of running with so many people had totally worn off. We were back down-town. My knees were feeling sore, my was breathing heavy, and my feet were starting to ache. I could feel myself slowing down and thought it would be okay if the Pace Keeper caught me. I'd still finish in the time I wanted, even if he did.

But then I heard screaming. I was worried there was another injury. But the screaming resolved into words. And the words . . . were my name. And it was my Juney!

"UNCLE   COOOOONNORRRRR!!!!" she screamed at the top of her little lungs. And there they were: Levi, Erin, Juney, and Clover. All at the street corner with a crazy, colorful, glitter-filled sign that read "Go, Connor, Go!"

"JUNEY!" I yelled back. "You're here!!" I yelled to them all. I ran over to their side of the street and tried to pause and hug them all, but they pushed me away.

"You're gross! Get moving!" Levi yelled at me. I mean, yes, I was super sweaty. I was gross. And so I did get moving.

"Love you guys!" I yelled over my shoulder.

My family was the encouragement I needed. My pace picked up, and I guess I caught a third wind. I had less than three miles left. I could do three miles. I did three miles all the time. I pictured my normal route from my patio: where the building was and where the downhills were, the curves in the trail. I could get there. I could do this.

The end of the race was on the other side of the starting line. We were running a huge loop around the city. I could hear music, crowd noise, and the announcer on loudspeaker saying things like, "Here comes number 364! Finish strong! We've got Mindy, number 273, coming up next. Great job, Mindy!" I turned a corner and could see the end, and I just sped up with no thought. I was charging as fast as I could toward that finish line, head down, legs pumping, arms swinging fast. The announcer yelled, "Here's Connor coming in hot! Great job, Connor!" My thighs were screaming and my head was roaring with excitement for being done, for finishing with excellence. The clock above the finish wasn't just under two hours. It was under an hour and fifty minutes. My final time was 1:43:50!

Once across the line, I stumbled a bit but kept moving. Someone put a finisher's medal over my head, and someone else gave me one of those silver blankets. I didn't need it, and I didn't see either of their faces. I was astonished and numb. The race was finished, and I had done better than I had ever hoped.

And suddenly Leah was there! She was hugging me and jumping up and down. I was kind of shaky and light-headed. I didn't really know what she was saying, but agreed with her enthusiasm. She took my picture, and I steered us to the tent with drinks and bananas.

After another few minutes, once I had some electrolytes in my system, I felt a lot better. I was so surprised to see Leah, especially that she had found me so quickly! Of course, she and Erin had been communicating about where I was on the route; I think the chip on my bib connected with a map in an app or something. Leah reported that they were taking us out to breakfast and were getting a table as we spoke. We walked around a bit longer to let my body cool down, and I did some stretches before getting into her car.

I felt so amazing the rest of the day and continued to get calls and texts from more people to find out how I did. My discipline had really paid off.

After picking up my car after breakfast, Leah came to my place to get the map to show Warren the next day. I felt its absence from my office, as if the place was emptier. The condo had felt this way when Pumpkin had to spend the night at the vet after getting neutered. It was a weird feeling. I took a long nap after my tradition of icing my feet.

38

THE PARK DISTRICT EXECUTIVE DIRECTOR

Connor Jackson

I t felt unnatural to go back to work the day after my race. I'd switched shifts with a coworker to get off on Wednesday for my court date, so I didn't want to push it and swap another day. I should have requested the day off long before. As ever, my feet ached and so did my quads, but my spirit was still uplifted. I took the entire week off from running. Erin and Leah were really trying to get me to come to another spinning class, but I shrugged them off. Spinning was definitely not my exercise of choice. I thought I'd swim at the rec center one day, at the most.

Al was really sick, as expected, and slept most of the day. His closest neighbor was on her fourth day of chemo. Everyone was pretty calm. My coworkers all wanted to hear about how I both nursed a guy with a twisted ankle mid-race and blasted my expected finish time. I was proud to tell the story more than once.

After lunch, Leah texted to ask if I could talk for a few minutes. She had news.

I found myself again in a family conference room. She tried to do her small talk with me before getting to the point.

"So how are you feeling today, Mr. Half-Marathon? Any sore muscles?" she said, her voice teasing.

"Yeah, I'm sore today, but not complaining. You're killing me here! What's the news?"

"Okay, okay, the Park District executive director, Alice Fitzgerald, paid me a visit this morning. She came with Warren to see the map."

"Whoa. The big boss lady in person, huh?"

"Yeah, it's not like she visits golf courses very often. I was not expecting her!" Leah sounded a little exasperated. "But she wanted to tell me face-to-face that she likes the historical significance of the building. She wanted to see it in person."

"Likes the significance of our building!" I exclaimed.

"It won't get torn down!"

"This is awesome! What great news!" And again I found myself excitedly jumping around in the family conference room.

"She wants me to work with the education team to draft some interpretive signage, and even put up some information about it in the golf clubhouse. We're supposed to talk with the American Underground Railroad History Museum and Research Center to make sure it's accurate. They also want to provide information about how it was a sugar shack and then how the Park District used it afterward. It really has a storied history."

"This is so great! I can't believe it!" I said.

"Totally! So I went and showed them both the building and Alice took down the police tape herself. I asked her about the people at the council meeting, and she said that they did not understand its entire history; they were only concerned about one week in its history. She was not worried about them at all. Warren, of course, is on board with keeping it up and is going to talk to Ralph about how to take down the fence but not the building."

"Yeah. The fence and not the building. Cool. What a turnaround!"

"And, Connor, he loves the map. He's really confident that the local historical society museum will accept it. But I think it's going to be harder than we thought to really give it to someone else, to part with it. Do you, like, want to say goodbye?"

I let out a sigh and paused before answering. "It is really weird knowing it's at your golf clubhouse and not in my office on top of the filing cabinet."

"I thought you'd feel that way."

"Being in a museum will be even weirder," I said slowly.

"Yeah."

After a moment, I said: "Do you think they could make me a copy?" She made a noise in the affirmative. "And they'd make some signage in the historical society museum, too, right? Maybe they could mention that you and I found it?"

"I bet they would. I'd really like that."

39

THE VISIT

Katie Brandt

About a month after I got out of the hospital, I decided I was well enough for a short walk on a trail, a walk on a very specific trail. I really needed to see that building! Travis and I packed up the kids in our black minivan with pink stickers on the back window and drove about an hour to Connor's home. He told me it was the first time he had ever hosted a former patient and their family. I'm fine to be a first in that department. Leah was there, too. It was so nice to meet her in person after talking to her on the phone and then hearing so much about her from Connor. She was lovely. They both took turns running around after PJ while Travis pushed the girls in our double stroller. I had forgotten that the trail from Connor's house was mostly uphill to the building. I was more winded than anyone else, but that just goes with the territory when you're recovering from obliterating your immune system.

When we arrived, Connor gushed over how it had changed since that first time he noticed the door being ajar. That first conversation we had about the structure felt like a lifetime ago. The surrounding fence was gone. You could see where the fence posts had been taken out, filled in, and reseeded with grass. The grass was still growing between bits of straw. The door had been permanently removed. Apparently, that will deter vandals. Unfortunately, the trapdoor was locked. Leah said that the local historical society now holds the map, a unique artifact that shows off Hawthorn Heights's formerly unknown involvement with the Underground Railroad. Connor showed off the framed copy hanging in his dining room.

I felt so proud when I visited the building. It was wonderful to see it in person instead of on a screen. The brick was warm to my touch, and the building was everything I expected and more. We had helped spare this little building. It was going to educate people about the town's history, the Underground Railroad, and even how maple syrup was made. It was going to be okay, and so was I.

40

THE ENDING

Connor Jackson

S pinning Leah and I are engaged now. I proposed during a late-night walk on our trail after the signs went up next to our historic building. She's been boxing up her stuff and slowly moving it into my place. Her deck furniture is way better than what was on my patio. The wedding is set for next September. There will be two flower girls in the wedding who couldn't be more excited.

We both had court hearings for our late-night illegal visit to the sugar shack turned runaway-slave shelter turned shortwave radio repeater station. I sat mostly silent during my time in court, since I did not want to tell the judge that I didn't regret my actions. Since Leah and I provided evidence that the building had a lot of significance, we got off with no community service requirements but did receive misdemeanors and fines. So now both of us have criminal records. Technically. I'm okay with that. The mob of angry villagers was right, it seems.

Leah has started running with me a bit. We're planning to do a 5K together in the spring. I've decided to do a triathlon next summer, too, which will incorporate running, swimming—and cycling. I'm not sure if another half is in my future or not. I'm thrilled with my personal best time and feel like that conquest was completed. That's certainly not to say I'm done with running. My disenchantment with the sport was short-lived, and I'm still on the trail at least four times a week.

Katie is doing great, almost half a year later. Her little girls are small but mighty, hitting all milestones when they should. Katie herself is still recovering, which is normal. Her hair is growing back, but she tires easily. Winning the war against cancer takes nearly everything out of anyone in the fight, and it did for her. I love that we still keep in touch and am honored to be her friend. Katie and Travis already told us they'll be at the wedding, even though invitations haven't been sent out yet.

ACKNOWLEDGMENTS

Always, thank you to my supporting and loving husband, Nate. I could never author books without his emotional backing (and wouldn't want to do life without him, either). Thanks to our son, who considered me to be an author long before I had any published books. Many thanks to my sister Meg, whose story and life inspired most of this manuscript, and to my mom, Linda, who believes all of her daughters have magical powers and can do anything they want, including publish books.

I appreciate all the cheerleading, ideas, and fact-checking from my many beta readers, some so early they may not recognize this manuscript: Meg and Linda, along with Marissa, Erin, Peg, Rene, and Heather, plus ladies from my local Facebook running group: Amanda, Tina, Jennifer, and Sara. Thank you all so much!

Thanks to Al for telling me the real story of the building near our house similar to this one, Erin for knowing legal stuff, Geoff for golf course info, David for telling me what it's really like to run a half-marathon, and Joe for his constant writing encouragement.

I also appreciate all the knowledge downloads and support from Write Publish Sell, Dallas Woodburn, and my Poison Pen writing ladies. Thanks to my first editor for all her ideas, Alyssa, and to my current editor, Beth. My words always need an editor's eyes!

Author's Notes

We grew up in a town steeped in history about the Underground Railroad. It was a joy to do some more research on the subject. That being said, I knew nothing about HAM radios or making maple syrup before starting this manuscript, but enjoyed reading about both. I used to work in watershed restoration and so had to reign in my watershed education dialogue. Thanks to the readers who didn't roll their eyes during the conversation Connor had with Richard!

I made up many of the locations in this book but based them on real places, with the exception of the Buckeye Trail. I highly recommend the hiking path! The American Underground Railroad History Museum and Research Center is not a real place but is based on the National Underground Railroad Freedom Center in Cincinnati.

I'd also like to write a special note to anyone dealing with cancer and stem cell replacement procedures. I hope you have nurses as wonderful as my sister had. You will make it to the other side, but it will take a lot out of you. Like Katie (and Meg), breaking your immune system down to build it back up is hard, so hard, but worth it. I wish you all the best and send as much encouragement and love as I can through time and space.

ABOUT THE AUTHOR

Iris March grew up the oldest of three sisters whose names all began with the same letter. Her sisters are still her best friends. March works in the sustainability field and also writes cozy mysteries in the Succulent Sleuth series. She lives in Ohio with her husband, young son, and three cats.

CPSIA information can be obtained
at www.ICGtesting.com
Printed in the USA
LVHW040325080922
727813LV00005B/240